TOMCATS & HOUSE CALLS

TOMCATS &
HOUSE CALLS

memoir of a

COUNTRY DOCTOR

WILLIAM O'FLAHERTY, MD

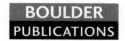

BOULDER
PUBLICATIONS

LIBRARY AND ARCHIVES CANADA CATALOGUING IN PUBLICATION

© 2012
O'Flaherty, William
Tomcats and house calls : memoir of a country doctor / William
O'Flaherty.

ISBN 978-1-927099-10-0

1. O'Flaherty, William. 2. Physicians--New Brunswick--Biography. 3. Physicians-
-Newfoundland and Labrador--Biography. 4. Medicine, Rural--Atlantic Provinces--
Anecdotes. I. Title.

R464.O45A3 2012   610.92   C2012-901266-1

Newfoundland
Labrador

We acknowledge the financial support of the Government of Newfoundland and
Labrador through the Department of Tourism, Culture and Recreation.

Canada

We acknowledge the financial support for our publishing program by the Government
of Canada and the Department of Canadian Heritage through the Canada Book Fund.

Published by Boulder Publications
Portugal Cove-St. Philip's, Newfoundland and Labrador
www.boulderpublications.ca

Editor: Stephanie Porter
Copy editor: Iona Bulgin
Cover design and page layout: Alison Carr
Front cover photos: lab coat, istock © dra_schwartz; caplin, istock © Segiy Gouppa
Back cover photo: istock © Stephen Orsillo

Printed in Canada

To my paternal grandparents,

William O'Flaherty,
who died before I was born,

and

Mary O'Flaherty (Granny),
who worked diligently helping to raise
her grandchildren in Long Beach.

This book is a product of more than 40 years of dealing with people in two provinces, interactions that numbered in the tens of thousands.

To protect the people mentioned in this book, names and identifying characteristics have been altered.

TABLE *of* CONTENTS

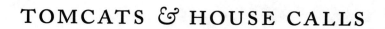

TOMCATS & HOUSE CALLS

MILK FEVER

"MY SON, THE COW IS PERISHING."

I suppose all of us who have practiced medicine in a country setting have had to deal, at one time or another, with sick animals. With the nearest veterinarian 100 miles away, difficulties with winter travel, and simple lack of finances, the nearest helping hand was called upon — and we responded, albeit reluctantly.

My first exposure to veterinary problems was not as a practicing country doctor, however, but as a child in rural Newfoundland.

My father spent a great deal of his life away from home, earning a living in various places to supplement sometimes meagre earnings from the cod fishery. At these times, my mother had the full responsibility of caring for a growing family of six children, my elderly grandmother, and a stable full of cattle. "Cattle" meant sheep, horses, cows, and hens — and this livestock resource was an important part of life. In those days we lived off the land and depended on our animals for milk, meat, eggs, and wool.

On that March day, when I was 12 years old, I immediately realized the depth of concern in my mother's voice: "My son, the cow is perishing."

The cow had calved two days before, and my mother had gone to the barn to milk her. She found the animal lying on her side, unresponsive but still alive. Around her were broken boards from the sides of the stall, evidence of struggle during the night.

My mother had dealt with various family cows during the years she was rearing her brood, and she felt an empathy and compassion for them that only mothers feel for one another. Her distress at finding her family cow at the point of death was not only because of the potential loss of a family resource but also because of affection for the animal. My mother was always the one who milked the cow. She accepted it, and the cow expected it. My father tried to milk her once or twice, and swore off that activity forever.

"Jane," he said, "damned if I'm going near that cow again. The next time she'll kick the guts out of me."

"Oh for God's sake, Gus," replied my mother. "It's only because of those hard old hands you got."

On this particular morning, my father was away at the seal fishery and not expected home for weeks. My mother said to me, "My son, go up and get Mullaly and bring him down. He's good at this kind of thing, they say."

Up I went, a mile up the snow-covered dirt road. Mullaly was home, and I told him the problem. "The cow is down and she can't get up and the calf is bawlin' and blarin' with the hunger."

"I got to get McCarthy to help out with this business," he said.

Neither of them had any particular expertise or training in veterinary affairs. They were just older members of the community who had a reputation for having some experience with illness in animals, and, like everybody in those days, they were willing to help out as best they could when called upon.

Mullaly, McCarthy, and I went back down the road, with the two of them questioning me: "Did your mother give that cow any frosty potatoes? What about the afterbirth?"

To the first question I answered, "no"; to the second, "I don't know," because I didn't know what they were talking about in the first place.

In the stable, my mother admitted giving the cow potatoes but not frosty ones. And she hadn't seen any afterbirth.

"She ate it," stated McCarthy.

"Or it's still inside her," declared Mullaly.

"Both ways, that's bad," said McCarthy.

Next came warm water, Sunlight soap, and Mullaly's arm, duly washed, up inside the cow.

"Nothing in there," he said.

"Poor hopes," predicted McCarthy.

They put their heads together and consulted, while my mother and I looked on.

"My son," they said to me, "go up to March's and get 10 packs of Epsom salts."

"Ten packs?" my mother, incredulous, asked.

"Ten packs," they repeated.

Up I went again, a mile and a half to a local store, and down again with the salts.

They took a rum bottle, wound the mouth of the bottle round and round with adhesive tape ("sticking plaster"), then filled it up with the Epsom salts solution and pushed it down the animal's throat, holding her head up so that most of it went down where it was supposed to.

"Now then, we'll see," Mullaly uttered, more to himself than to the rest of us.

Two hours passed, and the morning wore on into the early afternoon. The cow was still down.

"Jane," they announced, "I think she's finished."

Just then Woodfine came into the barn. He had heard about O'Flaherty's cow.

The three of them put their heads together.

"Jane, we think she needs some spirits o' nitre."

My mother looked at me, sad-like, and said dejectedly, "Boy, go up to March's and get some."

Up the road I went again and brought back the spirits o' nitre, an unknown substance to me then, unknown to me now, but mentioned sometimes years ago as being given to horses when they had "stoppage o' water."

I suppose, in desperation, the trio wanted to give the dying cow something rather than nothing.

Down the throat of the cow went the spirits o' nitre.

It was now late afternoon and the cow was still down. We had given up all hope when Woodfine remarked, in an offhand way, "I hear tell Doyle, down there in Gull Island, had a cow like this last winter and Tucker from Burnt Point did something to her udder, and she didn't perish."

"My son," said my mother, "go down and get Tucker."

I went 2 miles down the road and told Tucker what was going on. He had a horse and sleigh, and on the way back he asked me what had been done to the cow.

"They went up inside her, and they gave her 10 packs of salts, and some spirits o' nitre."

He muttered "Blessed Jesus" under his breath so I wouldn't hear. He was Protestant, you see, and they weren't supposed to swear, not like us Catholics. I could let out a few big ones, even at age 12, when my father and mother were out of earshot.

He took one look at the cow, the broken stall boards, the bawlin' calf, and declared: "Jane, she got the milk fever."

None of us had heard the like of this before. I can't say we disbelieved him. Let's just say we took the man's word with a grain of salt, taking into account that his area of expertise was not veterinary medicine but rather with the Newfoundland Light and Power or whatever it was called in those days. He was known as the "light man."

"Jane, I got to pump up her udder."

The other three, after a hurried conference, agreed, under one condition: they would go along with the proposed method of treatment provided she was given more Epsom salts as well.

Well, Tucker was having none of it. He gathered up his gear, and started out the door. "I'm having nothing further to do here."

My mother stood up, tall and firm, and said, "Mr. Tucker, sir, she'll be given no more Epsom salts. You do whatever you have to do and God bless you. Gus is at the seal fishery, and I'm the one to make decisions here, along with that bedlamer boy."

He went to work, inserting a metal tube into each teat and pumping up each quadrant of her udder, tying torn straps of cloth around each teat to keep the air from escaping.

"And now," my mother said, "come into the house and have a bite o' supper, all four of ye, that Granny has got ready. We can't do any more here. If she lives, she lives; if she perishes, she perishes."

One hour later, when we went out to the barn, the cow was up, bawling to the calf in another stall. Off came the cloth strips and in came the calf, starving after a 24-hour fast, not caring that what went down its gullet was half air and half milk.

Years later, when I went back as a family doctor to practice in the area where I was born, I had a family cow, a Jersey, that developed milk fever. Then I knew all the medical words I needed. I knew the pathophysiology of its condition — calcium from the mother's body pours into her milk, leaving her in a state of hypocalcemic tetany. It was easy for me to set up an intravenous calcium solution and help the cow back to a normal state. The recovery of the Jersey was routine, rapid, and expected.

But back then, a miracle of sorts, in the estimation of all of us, had occurred. The heroics in the story belong to the four men involved, to my mother, and, I suppose, to the 12-year-old who walked his legs off that day to save the family cow.

the OLD STORYTELLER

I HAD JUST ARRIVED on the shore — the new doctor, fresh from a seven-year stint working in hospitals in St. John's. The voice on the phone sounded hesitant and worried.

"I'm wanting some pain pills for Jackie. He's got that sciatic again, worse this time. Awake all night with the misery. Pain down his leg, same as before. I'll send up the young fella."

I knew the family; I had grown up in the area and re-membered the "old fella" Jackie, a storyteller who enthralled us young boys about days gone by when all the world was young. He was a thin little man with a moustache and a beard that always needed trimming. He lived off some sort of long-term government handout and always appeared to be happy and content with whatever the fates threw his way. His son, the "young fella," followed in his father's foot-steps and was a stay-at-home who accepted his lot in life of caring for his elderly parents. He was away from home just once, for 10 days during which he worked as a pick and shovel labourer in St. John's. Ten days of that was enough for him. He returned to Herring Cove, never again to leave the sheltered existence that was readily available for him on the North Shore.

The arrival of a new doctor in an outport community in Newfoundland is an event that is often looked upon as the highlight of the day and sometimes the news of the month. After all, you may need him tomorrow. You are certainly going to need him sometime — him and the clergyman, unless of course you feel that the services of the latter gentleman would be needed only when the ministra-tions of the former have failed miserably. The doctor is there, sir, and you'd be wise to look him over.

In the first few weeks of practice, the new doctor is scrutinized and discussed ad nauseam. People who have an appointment are questioned about the doctor's various and sundry qualities, especially "if what he gave you for what ails you cured your complaint." The physician in those first few weeks — first impressions being what they are — lays the groundwork for ongoing success or dismal failure. One mistake, or what is perceived as a mistake, in those first weeks, and his future is in jeopardy.

I asked the wife of my old storyteller, the man with the bad leg and the diagnosis of sciatica — which was her diagnosis, his diagnosis, the son's diagnosis — if he could walk.

"Oh no, Doctor, his leg is right paralyzed," she replied. "Paralyzed just like before when he got the sciatic. The young fella gets the sciatic too, every now and then. Runs in the family. We had the preacher up a couple of days ago, just before you got here, and he prayed over Jackie, and over me too, and told me the Lord would cure all ills, including the sciatic. I think a few pain pills, so he can get some sleep and, you watch, he'll be as good as new."

I was swamped with calls those first few days in the practice. The people had anticipated my arrival and put off visits to out-of-area physicians for problems that were not urgent. Their symptoms took time to sort out, especially since all of them were new to me, many with complicated and multiple complaints. When the son arrived at the clinic door, it was tempting to give him some medication for his father, let it go at that, short-term, and make a house call in a couple of days to follow up.

I spoke to the son, the young fella.

"Your father's not well, I hear; bad leg, eh? In the bed."

"Yis, b'y. Laid up pretty bad. Shockin' bad pain in the leg. Preacher said he'd be better be this time. Gettin' worse he is. Gettin' worse. An' he with the diabetes."

I had never attended him as a family doctor. My only contact with him was as a boy, sitting in his 100-year-old house, listening to his tales of his boyhood when the men from Herring Cove went off to "fight the Hun."

And now I was his family doctor.

"I'm going down to see him," I said to Cal, the son.

He looked surprised but said nothing.

When I arrived at the home, I could sense the aura and the smell of impending death. You get that only in the home of a dying person. You never notice it in hospital wards, blotted out, as it is, by disinfectants and alcohol swabs and deodorants. In the home it hits you full in the face.

His pulse was thin and rapid. His blood pressure was significantly below normal. He was lucid, but just. The leg all the way down from the hip to the toes was black and cold. Terminal gangrene.

He recognized me. "How are ya, b'y?" he asked. Just like old times.

I spoke to the wife and the son. I told them what I was about to tell our old storyteller.

"You're dying, Jackie. You have gangrene and the poison

has spread to your kidneys and your heart. There is a faint chance, if amputation is performed in the hospital, that your life may be saved. But I don't think so."

"Give me something for pain. Dats all I want. I'll die in me bed. Do dat and you're a grand young fella, dat's what you are."

I gave him an injection of Demerol, 50 milligrams, in his good hip and waited there by the bed where he had lain for days until he went to sleep, finally relieved of his pain.

He didn't wake up.

He was one of my first patients after I left the city to go out into the country practice. Out there, without the massive support offered by modern hospitalization, you cope as best you can. You deal with the hopelessly ill, the incurable, and the dying. At the end of life, when all hope is gone, most want to die at home, in familiar surroundings with family and friends all around. In those circumstances they die with dignity, always appreciative of every little gesture of kindness and every little item of care.

the MAN *from* HIGH POINT

OUR MAN FROM HIGH POINT began fishing in Ochre Pit Cove, up the shore a ways, when the government constructed a new wharf and an enlarged fishing stage there. Maybe more important than the wharf, actually, was the fact that he had a brand new pickup truck, the type the people of the Miramichi in New Brunswick call a half-ton: he could now drive up the shore, every day, to where his small punt was anchored inside the breakwater.

Our man was 60-something years old, his wife dead, and no family around. The only creatures that were close to him were his horse, used to haul firewood in the winter, and a female cat. He had adopted the cat as a tiny kitten; the mother had been run over by a car three or four days after she delivered the little beast. He reared the kitten on a concoction of Carnation milk and vegetable oil, and, as expected, the animal attached herself solidly to him as she thrived and grew. She even accompanied him up the shore half the time, staying in the cab of the pickup parked on the wharf while he was on the water.

He was familiar with the fishing grounds offshore Ochre Pit Cove, having steamed up there occasionally when the fish got scarce off High Point. He often gave advice to the younger fishermen: "Put Peg's Tolt between the spires of the church in Long Beach, and open up, just a little bit, the spire of the church in Broad Cove. You got that, me son? That's Little Bank. Nice drop o' water there though; 20 fathoms or so; hard to get the jigger down, sometimes, when she's runnin' a tide."

He would then describe, with great accuracy, the markings of other offshore fishing grounds — the Southwest Shoal, Howell's Bank, Nellie's Ledge, and The Grunt, the last one offshore Long Beach.

After an early morning spent jigging fish or hauling his trawls, he would come into Ochre Pit Cove, clear away the fish, and sell it green to the buyer there, saving a fish ("a nice black one," he always said) to cook for his dinner. It was the same meal, day after day, cooked on his Coleman stove on the tailboard of his truck. Into an old black bake-pot would go fat-back pork and onions, followed by the chopped-up fish and a couple of potatoes. A cup of salt water in there and a half-hour later the meal was ready. Not manna, but pretty close, my friend; pretty damn close indeed. And, of course, a nice bit of fish for the cat, which wasn't fussy whether it was cooked or raw.

Our man from High Point was well respected by the local fishermen because he generally caught more fish than they did — but also because he had the magic touch when it came to fixing the one-cylinder engines they all used in their boats. He was called upon most often in the spring, after the engines had been lying up all winter and were particularly stubborn in getting started. The fishermen, most of them jacks of all trades, had no problem solving most engine troubles but, occasionally, when the damn machines would die altogether, foul oaths would rain down on top of the things. One particular individual (who had bought his engine second-hand on a visit to Bonavista Bay) was particularly colourful with his curses, juiced up as they were with alliteration: "Bonavista Bastard!" he would shout (you could hear him out on the Rump, half a mile offshore). "Perlican Prick!" was another one, when he was particularly frustrated.

Our man would attend the stubborn engine and, with a few adjustments here and there, a drop of gasoline into the cup, a heave on the heavy flywheel, and bingo!, away she'd go more often than not.

You can see why he was so well respected.

But all was not sweetness and light. There was a problem.

As a small boy, our man was afflicted by "the Fever," as he called it, specifically rheumatic fever, and it left him with a damaged valve in his heart. It didn't affect his physical abilities when he was younger — a bit of swelling of the ankles, mild shortness of breath, occasional "beating" in the chest — but as he got older, he noticed that his shortness of breath was getting worse, and night brought spasms of coughing and persistent wheezing. The medication given to him by St. John's specialists was increased and "puffers" added, but were ineffective, other than providing some temporary relief.

He began to worry that the exertion of fishing was making his heart worse, and he expressed that concern when he was sent back for assessment by the specialists at the hospital in St. John's.

Several days later he visited me, his family doctor. Almost in tears, he said his condition was worse, and that he had been advised to stop fishing altogether.

"They have given up on me."

He was a religious man. Having lost hope of help from

mortals, he decided to seek divine intervention by visiting Brother Andre's shrine on the western side of the Mount Royal in Montreal. There, it is said, miracles have been bestowed on the faithful in abundance.

Off he went. He was in Montreal for a week and visited the shrine daily.

He came to see me on his return. He felt much better; as soon as he had arrived at the shrine, he had begun to improve. His wheezing, his cough, and his shortness of breath had practically disappeared.

He had no doubt that a miracle had occurred.

Ten days later he returned for a follow-up visit. To the sorrow of both patient and physician, he reported that all his symptoms had recurred, worse than ever. "In fact now, Doc, I can hardly get out of the house, pankin' for breath. I spends most of the time lyin' on the settle with the cat."

He refused hospitalization, despite efforts by the doctor and his neighbours in High Point to persuade him.

"Nothin' can help me now," he stated. "You know, Doc, all my life, the best I felt was when I was out there, on the water, hand-linin' the fish. I wish, one more time, I could get out to the Sou'west Shoal. One more time!"

It seemed he had given up on living.

Another fisherman from Ochre Pit Cove, he of the

colourful oaths and also a patient at the clinic, informed me several days later that he had visited our man in High Point and found him very upset. A neighbour's pit bull had killed his cat the day before.

"He was wishin' be the Lord Jumpin' Jesus that he could get out and get at that bloody bastard. He'd make short work of that dog. But ya know, Doc, he could hardly walk, he was pankin' for breath that much."

About a week later, on a trip down to the local cottage hospital, I had to pass by High Point on the way along and I decided to pay the man a visit. There were two reasons to do so — first, to check on his condition and, second, knowing how attached he was to the cat, to express some sorrow about the event.

He was out in the yard cutting up firewood. After an initial greeting, our man started immediately telling about the cat's demise.

"I let her out for one minute, Doc, and the pit bull jumped over the fence and was on her, broke her back in one second. She couldn't move her hind legs. And then he finished her off. But, Doc, she got her licks in before she went. She got her claws in an' tore the front off one of his eyes, right off, with the jelly-lookin' stuff runnin' out through the hole down the side of his face, down the fur on the side of his face. And he yelpin' and pawin' at his head on that side, an' goin' round in a circle an' bangin' into things.

"An you know, Doc, the next day and the day after that, his eye, or what was left of it, got all full of pus and the side of his face all swoll up, and the son of a bitch went downhill from there on. They shot him yesterday, to put him out of his misery. My cat died, Doc, but she took him with her! And damn good riddance, I say."

He was so animated in his description of the demise of his cat that he paid no attention to his own problems.

But I was paying more heed to my patient than to the story of the cat and was struck by the change that had occurred since I last saw him.

"You're a lot better since I last saw you. What's after happenin'?"

To be sure, the patient looked better, moved around without difficulty, with no signs of wheezing or coughing.

"You know, Doc, I tell you. I can't explain what it's all about, but right away, I swear to God, I got better after the cat got killed. I felt pretty bad about the cat, but the cough and the spit and all started to get better, and then you know what, the woman I'm talkin' to, over here from Old Perlican she is, came and cleaned out the place, washed it all, hung it out there on the clothesline, and that's when I really got better. I'm a new man. Yes, my son, I'm a new man."

The medical man from up the shore, trained in a top Canadian university, and his learned specialist colleagues in St. John's had all been wrong. All had failed to remember that common things are common and that a man incapacitated by an allergy to cats could suffer so severely and so long without recognizing the cause.

I owned up immediately.

"We were wrong. You have a heart condition, but your main problem was asthma brought on by an allergy to your cat. That's why you felt better in Montreal. That's why you improved when you went on the water."

Our man from High Point continued to gain strength. He soon resumed his previous activities including trips into the woods for firewood.

"Doc, you know what? I'm thinkin', next summer I might be able to get out to the Sou'west Shoal again. I still got the boat and the pickup, and now I got me health back, thanks be to God."

Yes, thank God all you want. And maybe, while you're at it, thank a certain pit bull as well; he gave you your health back, when the rest of us failed.

EMILY, JOSHUA, *and the* BLUEBERRY PIGS

BACK IN THE HARD TIMES in the Dirty Thirties, Emily and Joshua lived on the North Shore of Conception Bay. Although both were getting up in years at the time, Emily and Joshua, like everyone else on the Conception Bay North Shore, raised pigs. The people of that part of Newfoundland were called North Shore pork eaters, for good reason.

Emily and Joshua had two pigs: a boar and a sow. When the boar was still no bigger than a small dog, Joshua had called in the local horse doctor to castrate the wee beast. They did the deed by stuffing the pig, head first, down into a long rubber boot and going after the appropriate area with a red-hot iron.

Emily heard the racket in the yard and, being a religious

person and not wanting to see any of God's creatures bar-
barized, out she went and told the horse doctor, whom she
didn't like, to get the hell out of there and leave the fine
boar pig alone.

And thus, the intended result of the two men's endeav-
ours was left in doubt, in spite of the iron being very red
and very hot.

Emily, being the boss of the place, would have no truck
with any further business with the two pigs other than
feeding them boiled-up cod's heads and small potatoes,
like everybody else on the shore did.

When the fall of the year came round, the two pigs
were growing wonderfully well and putting on weight. The
two of them had half the backyard torn to pieces, as they
nosed their snouts into every bit of grass that could be
found. Emily, seeing this, said to Joshua: "My son" — you
can call every male on the North Shore "my son" — move
them two pigs in by the droke garden, 'cause the next thing
you know they'll be up under the house, glory be to God!"

And so it was in the late part of August Joshua built a
pen in the garden by the droke, a good ways in the woods
away from the house. He built it out of wattles, driving
some of them into the ground, and curling them onto three
longers, which were attached to the bushes.

He had a bit of trouble getting the pigs into the pen, because pigs are stubborn creatures, the worst God ever created, according to Emily. But with some help from a local giant of a fellow with more brawn than brains, and with a great din of squealing and cursing, the pigs were hauled into the new pen. Emily said that Joshua's soul was damned to hell in the process, for sure, what with all the swearing and cursing and taking God's name in vain.

During the late summer and early fall, Joshua fed the pigs their usual boiled cod's heads and small potatoes. The neighbours came around to tell Joshua what fine pigs they were and how they were sure to be great eating when the winter came. But Joshua noticed a strange thing: even though the pigs were healthy and growing, they never seemed to be interested in the food he threw into the trough each day. In fact, a couple of times he went in to check on them around duckish and found them stretched out asleep while the crows and gulls were having a grand time at the trough, eating up the works.

One day in early October, when the days were getting shorter and there was a bit of frost on the ground in the mornings, he went to feed his pigs, but they weren't in the pen. Not a sign of them anywhere. Gone. "Oh, my blessed God Almighty," he said to himself. "Somebody is after goin' off with me two fine pigs." And right away, out he went to Emily and told her about the terrible thing that had happened.

"'Tis no wonder, is it, what with all the cursin' and swearin' that went on," she said. "'Tis divine retribution taken hold, that's what it is. 'Tis not much pig pork we'll have this winter, we won't, and this being hard times and all, and what do ye expect, and ye takin' the name of the Lord in vain."

Well, back to the pen he goes, and lo and behold he sees the two pigs coming down over the hill, one behind the other, down over the hill behind the droke, marching right up to the pen, and crawling in through a hole beneath one of the longers. He saw that their chops and snouts were covered with blue juice and they had that colour on their trotters too.

Joshua realized that all through the late summer and fall the pigs were living on wild blueberries and herts, and all he was doing was feeding the crows and gulls on boiled cod's heads and small potatoes.

It wasn't long after that the cold nights got colder, and it was time to move the pigs from the pen above the droke into the pigsty in the barn close to the house. When that was done, the late fall was coming on fast. Soon it would be time to have a pig killing, like everybody else on the shore. One pig salted and stored in a barrel, and the other one quartered and hung up in the top cellar in the cold and frost, and a piece sawed off when a nice piece of pig pork was wanted.

Now one day, just before the time came for killing the pigs, the priest came for his annual visit, as he did for all houses in the parish. He came to collect his dues, to see how well off his people were, and to bless the house and the hay in the barn with holy water to make sure it didn't catch fire in the winter.

"Father O'Leary," Emily said, "I'm glad you came right about now. Me poor husband Joshua is laid up with a bad foot, the gout I think it is, and I want you to bless his foot, and the hay in the barn too. There's nothin' in the barn now except two pigs. The cattle are all out on the land, chewin' on the hummocks, so it won't be too crowded in there when you goes in to bless the hay."

Father O'Leary went out alone and blessed the hay. He knew the barn well, having been there several times before, and didn't expect Joshua to accompany him, what with his bad foot.

He came in and said, "Emily, I blessed the hay, and the two fine pigs you got as well. But I don't think, Emily, that you'll be killing two pigs for your winter pork. Maybe one, not the two of them."

"And why not, Father?" she asked.

"Because they were copulating in the pen when I was there."

"Copulatin'? What's that?"

"Havin' sex," the priest said.

"Oh my blessed Jesus in the manger!" she screeched. "That boar pig was done back in the spring of the year. He was done by the horse doctor with a red-hot iron!"

"I guess, Emily, it didn't work."

After he had gone, Emily and Joshua had a talk, with Emily doing most of the talking.

"How in God's name are we going to kill them two pigs, what with one of them being with young, and the two of them blessed by the hand of God? How are we goin' to do it a'tall, a'tall, after he blessin' them and all we wanted was for himself to bless the hay?"

They thought it over for awhile, with Joshua doing the thinking, and Emily still doing the talking.

"Joshua, we can't kill them two pigs. And we can't feed them this winter. Joshua, there's only one thing to do. We haven't been able to pay our dues for nigh on five year, what with the bad times upon us. We'll give the pigs to the priest, and he can do with them whatever he wants. He's got a nice big barn back of the church with an American horse and a Jersey cow. A couple of pigs would be welcome, I expect, especially ones that can be fed as easily as them two."

And so Emily and Joshua paid their dues. Each year after that, for quite a long time, Father O'Leary gave them two small pigs out of the yearly litter produced by the two blueberry pigs, so that the two old folks could have lots of pig pork to eat winter after winter.

NO SICK SOUP *for* LIGE

"DOC, I FEEL SO GODDAMN BAD TODAY I can smell the pine boards."

And that was my introduction to the man. We will call him Elijah, or "Lige," as they say on the North Shore.

He was in his 60s and lived alone in a small outport house in a small community on the shore. His wife had died years before. His only son had gone away to the war as a soldier. The son had survived the conflict and married an English girl — and there he stayed, in Ipswich, England, living the life of an English countryman. He returned just once, on the death of his mother. After the funeral, he returned to England, knowing that the next time he would return to Newfoundland would be to attend another funeral. There was no other reason to visit. He was no longer a Newfoundlander; the North Shore was a distant memory.

Lige was an average rough and tumble outport person, living off the land and the sea, and completely self-reliant. He owned his home and his few acres of land, a barn in which he housed his mare, and a root cellar where he kept his potatoes and turnips during the winter. The mare was used to haul the firewood he cut on Crown land back of the community to burn in his wood stove.

When Lige came to my office for that first visit, he tried to joke about his symptoms. It is a fact, however, that some men, especially those who rarely visit the doctor's office, tend to minimize their complaints and often lie about them. The man was short of breath and had a hacking productive cough and a fever. There were signs of pneumonia in his left lung. He was so informed.

"Hospital," I said.

Silence. Dead air.

"I'm not goin'," Lige said.

In those days, in the minds of the North Shore people, hospitals were where you went to pass on into the next world. That was especially true when it came to dealing with the deadly disease of tuberculosis, or consumption, as it was called then. You went to the hospital and came out in a wooden casket.

Lige would have none of it.

"You treat me home, Doc, or else I'll go to me place and rub Vicks on me chest, and boil up some molasses and kerosene, and take me chances on it all. But I'm not goin' to the hospital."

I visited Lige at home over the next week, giving him daily injections of penicillin. Lige refused to accept more help in the form of visits from a public health nurse.

"You're the man," he said. "No one else comes in here." Lige's reluctance to have anybody enter his home, especially strangers, was understandable. Elderly men who live alone don't spend much time on such niceties as sweeping and dusting. Now that he was ill, the situation had further deteriorated, but it was still liveable. A woman, especially a nurse coming into his place and seeing the clutter, would have "taken over," Lige worried, and that would have been the end of his independence.

As his pneumonia improved over the week and he got back on his feet, Lige made a statement I would remember years later.

On the shore it is common practice for neighbours to bring food for the patient, relatives, and caretakers when sickness or death strikes a family. In the community where Lige lived that charity is called "sick soup."

On the last visit I made, when Lige was fully recovered, he said: "Doc, nobody will bring sick soup to Lige."

The years went by, and as Lige got older and reached the biblical quota of three score and ten, it became obvious he was becoming frailer. The common tasks that had become part of his life, such as planting his garden and harvesting the hay for his mare, were now more difficult. Going in the woods to cut firewood became impossible, and he had to buy firewood and coal for his stove. His mare became more of a pet than anything else. She had grown old along with her master. Finally, one morning, when Lige went out to feed her, he found her dead, her belly bloated, and the boards in her stall splintered from the death throes that had occurred during the night.

The last visit Lige made to my office was in his 76th year, one week before his birthday. He was still in reasonable health, other than the overall loss of strength and energy that occurs in most people of that age. He did have one new complaint. His vision was beginning to fail and he was experiencing pain in both eyes, enough to keep him awake at night. He had previously been diagnosed with mild glaucoma, which had responded to medication up to now.

"Doc," he said, "I don't want the man above to pull the plug on me yet. But if I lose me sight, I don't want to stay around."

He was sent off to the eye specialist immediately.

The next day he disappeared.

Two weeks went by. The son in Ipswich was contacted by the parish priest and informed that local authorities had entered the home to make sure the old man was not dead in his bed. He refused permission for any further entrance to the premises until he arrived from England.

Down the shore, miles below where the old man lived, there is a towering cliff on the edge of the ocean called Redlands for the colour of the rocks. There is a straight drop of 300 feet to the salt water, interrupted in a few places by ledges jutting out from the rock wall. Occasionally, especially in the spring of the year, sheep and goats feeding on the upper reaches of the cliff have been known to fall over and land on the ledges far below.

Two weeks after Lige consulted the eye specialist, some fishermen noticed something on one of those ledges. They presumed it was a small rock slide, or perhaps a dead animal. But, considering that a man from up the shore had disappeared two weeks previously, the authorities were notified.

The next day, Lige's body was hauled up by a fireman lowered down to the ledge. His broken body showed evidence of a severely fractured skull after falling 200 feet. Death had been swift, sudden, and painless.

When Lige's son came from England and searched the house, he found a typed note from the eye specialist directed to the family doctor, written on the day of the visit, stating that complete loss of vision could be expected in six to 12 months.

Lige's will left considerable money to the church. The son raised some legal objections, but the last testament was declared valid, and he went back to England, never to return.

The old man's house and land fell into disrepair, and soon, with the fences rotting and falling down, the property became part of the community commons.

Lige is remembered by his physician and his neighbours as a fiercely independent outport character who depended upon nobody but himself and died rather than become a burden to his fellow man.

the CLERGYMAN *and*
FILTHY LUCRE

IN SALMON GUT, on the North Shore of Conception Bay, there lived a man of the cloth, much beloved of God. He described the church grounds and buildings he lived in as "an oasis in a desert of desolation," the desert of desolation being the North Shore.

Our man grew up on a farm in the countryside of England. As a teenager, he was expected to do daily chores. One day, while helping the local veterinarian castrate a young stallion, the boy received a well-aimed kick from the unappreciative horse. The hoof caught the boy full force just below the left knee, an injury so severe that both bones were fractured, with the splintered fragments driven out through the skin.

Long months of recuperation followed. The young lad

occasionally hovered close to death, racked with fever from infection spreading from his leg to the rest of his body. Surgery was required to remove dead and infected bone; amputation was contemplated several times.

In those months while he lay in bed, he sometimes hallucinated for hours. During one of those periods, he was visited by a divine personage, an angel who promised his life would be spared if he would amend his sinful ways and become a Christian clergyman. He presumed the first visitation was a bad dream. After all, such illusions can occur under the influence of high fever, especially when pain-controlling medication is being used.

When the apparition returned a second time, however, the lad felt the matter needed addressing. He called in the local priest to discuss what was now a frightening turn of events. The priest, a man of great faith, advised him to agree to the conditions outlined by the heavenly apparition and to prepare himself for a life in the service of the Lord.

And so it was. Months after the initial injury, he emerged, emaciated but still alive, with a leg that had miraculously healed but was several inches shorter than the other. For the rest of his life, he walked with a noticeable limp. When he was finally able to hobble along on his own, arrangements were made by the priest for him to go to a seminary in Spain for theological training.

There, burdened by the formidable promise that would rule the rest of his days, he plunged wholeheartedly into the study of religion. He learned Latin, Spanish, the Scriptures, the philosophy of Thomas Aquinas and Augustine, the history of the Christian church, and, unfortunately, not much else. He learned enough, however, to regard himself as an authority on most matters affecting mankind. Such an attitude, regrettably, afflicts many clergymen — then, as now.

Upon finishing his theological training, he was ordained and became a curate with the priest who had advised him during his illness. Europe had an oversupply of Christian clergymen at that time and, when he went looking for a parish of his own, he found the pickings pretty slim. North America, on the other hand, what with great waves of immigration occurring at that time, was in dire need of religious leaders.

Not long afterward, our man sailed to Newfoundland and established himself on the North Shore of Conception Bay in a parish that had only been served by itinerant clergy up to then. Soon after he settled in, several members of his family immigrated to Newfoundland and tried to find work in the farming area south of St. John's. They quickly realized that farming in Newfoundland was not the same as farming in England and soon moved on, one to Prince Edward Island and three to the parish on the North Shore to help their priestly relative.

Our man's parish stretched along the coastline for many miles, and most of his flock came to the church in Salmon Gut for sermons and religious rituals. Many of the parishioners were poor fishermen who lived off the sea and the land and got by without needing large amounts of money.

But this clergyman did. He definitely needed, as he called it, "filthy lucre."

After all, he had the priest's house to run. In that house lived a host of unemployed relatives, including a cousin from Ireland reputed to be an atheist, who found it not at all unusual that he should live on parishioners' contributions to a religion that worshipped a supreme being whose very existence he denied. "I'll eat good Christian grub any day," he would say in his singsong Northern Ireland accent.

As well, there was a man from Angashore Bight, employed full-time to tend the wood and coal furnaces in the basements of the house and the church.

All that needed money.

So on Sundays and Holy Days, and the 40 days of Lent,

and other days as well, our man of the cloth gave fire-and-brimstone sermons predicting certain and imminent damnation, not because of sins against their Lord and Creator but rather because the collection plate wasn't filled to his liking. In great and thunderous tones, enough to shake the church, he would criticize parishioners for failing to pay their dues. He would rail against the paucity of the Sunday collections and the lack of support for missions, the Christmas collection, the Easter collection, the Lady Day collection, and maybe the collection for the "Lady of Low Point," or some other celestial and holy personage.

An entourage of altar boys attended our man during any service in the church: eight (or sometimes 10) lined up across the front of the altar. Two were servers. The rest were there for show. All were dressed in red soutanes and white surplices.

The altar boys were usually in their early teens, and youngsters in that age group are unpredictable in their behaviour. One of their duties was to bring the communion water, wine, and the unleavened Host to the church from the priest's house, where it had been prepared by the clergyman's sister. Under no circumstances, under pain of terrible retribution, were the Host and the wine to be tampered with.

Now, what better reason is there to sample a nice drop of sherry wine than to be told that, for sure, God's wrath would strike you dead if you did so? And it was, believe me, a very nice sherry wine, as all the altar boys learned.

During the ritual, the two servers approach the altar, one with a small beaker of water, the other wine, and pour some of each into the proffered chalice held by the priest. The one pouring the wine was often warned beforehand by his fellow altar boys: "My son, look a'here, you go easy on that wine, ya hear? You give him too much wine, buddy, and there's a trimmin' comin', and don't you forget it."

Invariably there was almost always a nice drop of wine left in the beaker, none of which, believe me, went back to the priest's house.

The altar boys, sometimes called acolytes, sat on each side of the altar during the sermons, facing the side walls of the church. In this position none of them had eye contact with anybody, but that didn't stop them from interacting with one another with whispers and suppressed giggles.

On a particularly warm Sunday one July, when the church was filled with people, many of them visitors from away, the priest lambasted the parishioners for the poor response to his request for more money, made the previous Sunday.

"'Tis a good thing we have a few people from away coming in here. Else the collection box would be empty."

And on and on.

One of the altar boys, who had been particularly well fed the night before with Jiggs' dinner — pease pudding, cabbage, and the lot — was having problems with gas. As the priest rambled on, the boy, sitting on the steps at the side of the altar, was afraid to "let go," just in case there was more to it than gas, you understand. He held on as long as he could, hoping the service would end and he could get some relief in the sacristy.

The priest was particularly upset that day because one of the parishioners, instead of the usual $10 fee for dues, had offered only $5.

"Take it or leave it. That's all I can afford," was the parishioner's attitude.

"Aha! No way!" the priest responded. "Let one get away with it, they'll all want to pay $5!"

He read out the list of parishioners who had paid their dues and was about to announce the names of those who had not. He paused for breath. A pregnant pause. For a few seconds' lapse in time, an unusual silence pervaded the church.

Suddenly the distressed acolyte let go a long, loud fart,

the sound of which, helped by the acoustics of the church, could be heard the length and breadth of the building.

It doesn't take very long, does it, for the sacred to descend to the level of the profane?

The effect upon the service was immediate. The altar boys burst into laughter. In the front pews, occupied by the merchant class of the community, there was shocked silence. Farther down the congregation the people, knowing only that the explosion had come from the general altar area, suspected that the good reverend himself was the gassy culprit. One of them remarked: "If we're not hearing thunder from one end, we're hearing it from the other."

The priest, having started the sermon in a particularly foul mood, gave up all hope that the congregation would pay attention to what he was saying, especially when he observed that some of the worshippers had joined the altar boys in open laughter. The whole business was sacrilegious, and he rapidly finished off the ritual and stormed off the altar in a rage.

I have already affronted your delicate sensibilities enough, so I shall refrain from further comment, other than to state that when the altar boys were questioned, all of them denied having caused the commotion and only admitted to the ensuing laughter. For that, the priest said, they were all, without a doubt, headed for hell's fire and damnation.

To do justice to the legions of stories about this man would require a book. One can only nibble at them in a story such as this. Before closing the subject, however, one more incident cries out to be related.

Our man of the cloth was in the habit of frequently calling out from the pulpit requests for members of the community to work on the church property. This, of course, was unpaid labour and was so named "free labour." He would say something like this: "Angashore Bight. Free labour on Wednesday. And come with your horses and box-carts."

One day a man from up the shore a ways was engaged in free labour, along with a few neighbours from the same community, clearing away leaves and debris after the winter — spring cleaning, in other words. This man was not well off, money-wise, as his clothes and footwear attested. That day the sole of one of his leather boots came undone and was hanging there, still partly attached. It flapped each time he moved, so that his walk was a series of goose steps as he lifted the affected foot high off the ground. The priest noticed this situation and said to him: "Look, my good man, you can't work like that."

The labourer expected to be sent home. He was mistaken. The priest reached into the pocket of his greatcoat and pulled out a roll of bills held together with rubber bands. The roll was big enough to choke a horse. The group of labourers, seeing this, expected that a charitable event was about to take place — namely a $10 or $20 donation to get a new pair of boots.

The reverend started pulling at the rubber bands on the roll of bills.

He handed one to the labourer. "Here, my son. Put that around your boot."

Back in England, the priest's brother had taken over the operation of the family farm. When he eventually died, he left the estate to his sibling in Newfoundland. Thereupon our man, by then into old age, immediately left for the countryside of his childhood. He entrusted the parish to a young curate, a young man born on the North Shore, and never returned to Newfoundland.

During his retirement, the priest was asked what he thought of the population who lived on the North Shore of Conception Bay.

"They are a very gentle people," he replied.

Coming from him, that was an enormous compliment.

ANGUS, *the* GENTLE GIANT

ON THE NORTH SHORE of Conception Bay during the early years of Newfoundland as a province of Canada, in a place called Angashore Bight, there lived a man of great strength. We'll call him Angus. A bachelor all his life, Angus lived a quiet existence in the small community, getting along well with everyone, being courteous to all.

Angus was solid muscle and bone, and for that reason, as well as for his quiet demeanour, he was well respected all along the shore. Tales of his physical powers are legion to this day: one often-recalled incident involves Angus lifting an 800-pound engine (used to power a trap skiff) out of the boat, all on his own. And, in an area of the world where the measure of a man's prowess is judged by how many policemen it would take to bring him in when the need arose, it was said Angus would require most of the RCMP contingent to do the job.

Fishing was, and to some extent still is, the lifeblood of the North Shore. The cod was once king. Back then, swarms of codfish would migrate close to the shoreline each spring and summer, feeding on caplin and other small fish, providing a livelihood to the local fishermen. There were unpredictable years, however, when few fish came to shore; the fishery would fail and some other form of employment would be needed to get by until the next spring.

It is in that sort of year that this story takes place.

I must digress here to relate some relevant features of life in the young province of Newfoundland. The great Joey Smallwood was in charge and, for a long period of time, acted like a king rather than a provincial premier. Great announcements galore came from his lips, and the closer we came to an election, the greater the predictions of wonderful government programs. Most of the highways in rural parts of the province were gravel roads at that time, and Joey took full advantage of the monetary largesse streaming out of Ottawa to launch, big time, into the task of paving every road and drung he could find — most often, as I said, before an election.

Back to Angus and our story. The fishery failed that

year, and many families were left to face a hard winter. The fall came and the men were preparing to go to the lumber-woods, to St. John's, or to Halifax to work on the docks. And then, lo and behold, heavy paving equipment appeared on the gravel road that wound its way down the shore from Carbonear. The paving crew set up headquarters in a gravel pit on that part of the shore called the Highlands, a good ways down the road from Angashore Bight.

You can imagine the talk in the community. First, the highway was about to be paved; second, there was an election in the offing; and third, there was going to be employment for the men.

Angus saw all this, and when the boss of the paving crew, a man from Upalong, called for men to work, Angus was the first in the lineup. He was told that men with families would be given first consideration, and then, and only then, would he be hired. He accepted this in his quiet respectful way and went home, still hopeful he would get a job.

Sure enough, one week later, as I made my house-call rounds and passed by the paving crew just starting to work on the highway in Angashore Bight, there was Angus up on top of the black smoky paving vehicle, with a shovel in his hand, doing whatever had to be done up there. Each day on my rounds I would stop and speak to the men, most of whom were my patients, and wave to Angus up there in the smoke and the heat.

Several weeks later, with the work only half completed, I saw there was a new worker in Angus's place, a young man, unknown to me. I stopped and asked the other men if Angus was ill. They said, no, he wasn't sick, that he had been laid off and the new worker was the nephew of the boss, also from Upalong.

I had the feeling, as I drove away, that the paving crew hadn't seen the last of Angus.

Late that afternoon, as I was returning home from my rounds, I saw, about a mile up the road from the gravel pit, several hundred yards ahead of me, the figure of a large man, weaving back and forth across the road, "taking both sides of 'er" as the North Shore men say. It was Angus. I had to stop the car. He came over to the open car window and it was quite obvious that he had had a few too many.

"Go home, Doc," he said.

"Angus," I said, "I'm trying to go home, man, but you're in the way ..."

He interrupted, not paying any attention to what I was saying. "Go home, Doc," he repeated. "Go home and get your instruments ready. I'm goin' down to the gravel pit to get me job back. An' if I don't, Doc, I'm sendin' you up half a dozen."

And off he went, weaving down the road.

I went to the office (my residence and my clinic were in the same government-owned building) and waited, expecting God-only-knows-what.

The hours passed. Nothing happened, other than the usual run-of-the-mill problems.

The next day I stopped as I met the paving crew. There, up in the smoke and the heat, waving happily to me, was Angus, back at his old job.

I waved back at him. I must confess the wave was not just a wave; it was much more. It was heartfelt salute.

ESAU *and* HIS
BIBLICAL DIET

THERE IS A SMALL FISHING VILLAGE on the North Shore of Conception Bay in which all the people live high up on the upper reaches of a cliff that towers 300 feet above the sea.

You might wonder how such a place could be a fishing village, considering its location high above the salt water, but the explanation is simple. A small river, which flows through the community, has cut a deep sloping gorge all the way down to the ocean, terminating in a small crescent-shaped beach. The local fishermen have created a path, half a mile long, down the side of the valley, leading to the sandy beach. Access to the ocean, and to their livelihood, is readily attainable to those who live high above the ocean.

Along the shore the sloping river valley and the beach are referred to as "the Droke."

Years ago, Esau, a man of great religious convictions, lived in the community. He lived alone, unmarried, in a house on a small patch of land inherited from his father.

Esau, who had a rudimentary education, had acquired the habit of reading any and all books he could get his hands on. He looked upon himself, as did everyone else in the community, as being self-educated.

But the area in which he was considered a true expert was in his knowledge of the Bible. Esau spent a great deal of his time reading the Bible. He knew the Scriptures intimately, all the way from Genesis to Revelation. The lessons and directions he gained from his reading guided his life and regulated his daily activities.

He was 50-plus years of age at the time and physically a very healthy person who rarely visited the local family doctor. Insomnia was his only complaint and, in spite of therapy, he rarely slept any more than three hours per night. The rest of the time, until dawn, he read the Bible. Truth be known, he spent many hours of daylight doing the same thing.

In contrast to the hard-working fishermen in the community, Esau was rarely seen in a fishing boat. He confined his activities to tending a small kitchen garden and reading books (mainly, as stated, the Bible). He got by on a small

monthly government handout from the Smallwood social-
ists who were in power at the time. This was during the
infancy of Newfoundland as a Canadian province.

The locals considered Esau a harmless eccentric. As
often happens in many rural communities, they tolerated
him and, in some ways, granted him a degree of grudging
respect.

His diet was rather bizarre in that he attempted to follow, as much as reasonable, the dietary habits documented
in the Bible. He avoided pork and pork products altogether
— and that, while living among the North Shore pork eaters. To satisfy the biblical directions that one should ingest
only meat from animals with a cloven hoof that chew the
cud, he was forced, whenever he craved meat, to eat goat,
lamb, or beef. Because of his chronically unemployed state,
however, he rarely ate meat at all and supplied his protein
requirements by eating fish.

For this purpose he had gotten two large second-hand
deep freezers from a local grocery that had gone out of
business. All summer long, even though he was not a fisherman himself, he visited the fishing stages down in the
Droke daily (sometimes twice a day) and collected fish
heads, tomcods discarded as too small by the fishermen,
and caplin. He also gathered cod livers, which, years before,

were collected and processed into cod liver oil but now discarded as offal. He froze all of these items in his ample freezers, enough to last him through the upcoming winter.

That fish, and the meagre supply of vegetables from his small kitchen garden, formed his diet.

As a result of Esau's diet and the physical activity involved in his frequent visits to the Droke on his only means of transportation — his legs — he maintained a slim body without an ounce of fat. This was in contrast to some of his neighbours, who frequently overate pork and fatty salt beef, and often developed the side effects of obesity — diabetes, heart disease, high blood pressure, and other unnamed afflictions. He had none of these problems and attributed his good health to divine favour bestowed upon him because of his unshakeable fidelity to the God of the Bible. The illness of his neighbours, in his estimation, no doubt resulted from the mediocrity of their faith in the Lord, and, in consequence, a lack of His benevolence in regard to their health.

Esau, like most, occasionally dealt with the two professionals in the area in which he lived. The local physician he saw hardly at all, and then only for his insomnia, which continued unabated. The clergymen — usually young and cutting their teeth in their chosen profession, often staying on the shore for just a short period of time — were of more interest to Esau. Whenever a new clergyman appeared on the scene, he was summoned to Esau's residence and tested on his knowledge of the Scriptures.

Esau would start out with an easy question.

"How about Mark 10:25; you know that one, Reverend? No? I'll tell you: It is easier for a camel to go through the eye of a needle, than for a rich man to enter into the kingdom of God."

The clergyman, generally knowledgeable about most aspects of his religion, was no match for Esau.

"How about Numbers 11:5; you know that one, Reverend? That's about Moses, out in the desert, gallivantin' around out there for 40 years, livin' on manna with some of his entourage wishin' they were back in Egypt so they could have a bit more variety to their grub, maybe a bit of garlic to spice it up. And that included Moses's wife, an Ethiopian. Did you know that, Reverend?"

The poor clergyman, up here from North Carolina to save Canadian souls, would be left floundering, not knowing what hit him.

One clergyman stayed on the shore for 18 months, much longer than usual, and got to know Esau fairly well. In fact, he felt obliged, because of concerns for his parishioner, to speak to the doctor about this odd man in their midst.

One of his concerns was the unkempt state of his residence. Esau, after all, lived alone and, as is often the case in such circumstances, his place was in a mess, the lurid details of which I will spare you. Needless to say, in Esau's value system, cleanliness was not up there next to godliness.

The clergyman's other concern was the smell of the place.

When Esau's door was opened, there ballooned out, full force in the face, a smell of cod liver oil and something else yet to be determined. The place reeked of it. Esau's clothes reeked of it, too, so much that when he went to church on a Sunday, people moved to another pew.

An explanation is in order. Because of Esau's limited supply of food, he ate roasted cod liver, fried on his wood stove, almost on a daily basis. The physician had never seen this before, other than once in an Acadian restaurant in Caraquet, New Brunswick. The clergyman, hailing from Romford, Maine, and having graduated from a university in New York City, had never heard of roasted cod liver. Chicken liver, yes. Cod liver, no. The roasted cod liver accounted for some of the unpleasant smell, but not all.

In keeping with the biblical road map of his diet, and the reference to garlic in the book of Numbers previously mentioned, Esau ate prodigious amounts of garlic every day. He felt that it was health promoting, as many people do, but more importantly, garlic was mentioned right there in Numbers 11, for all to see. What more reason do you want to eat the stuff with your cup of tea and donut in the morning? The fact that it made you and your humble abode smell to high heaven mattered little.

It is not known what eventually happened to Esau. The doctor moved on. The clergyman from Romford, Maine, who had stayed for 18 months, left the North Shore and took over a charge on the Great Northern Peninsula, where, for some reason, his faith was sorely challenged. He determined that all this was not for him and obtained gainful employment as a forest fire warden on top of one of those high towers looking out over the landscape in the woods of northern Ontario. Up there, you deal with your God only. Down on earth, you have to deal with the strange, the odd, and the unpredictable.

CIGARETTES *and* BINGO

I FIRST MET ANNIE as a patient when she arrived to live on the North Shore. She had been born on the south coast of Newfoundland, where she had spent most of her life. She was a tiny woman, about 5 feet in height, 60 years of age, unsophisticated, and almost illiterate. Her background, which she was quite open about, was one of grinding poverty. After her husband died, her children all but abandoned her, and she moved in with her unmarried and generally unemployed brother. That was right after the war, just before Confederation with Canada.

When her brother died, Annie became quite depressed and needed psychiatric treatment in St. John's, where she was hospitalized for a while. After discharge, Annie did not want to go back to the south coast. The hospital arranged for her to stay in a community hostel on the shore. It was one of these places designed to care for recuperating psychiatric patients after a stay in hospital. She lived in the hostel a year and then, having developed some friendships in the community and acquired a disability pension, she rented a small apartment in a low-cost complex built by a service organization for those in need.

Annie was reasonably content in this new arrangement and was able to stop taking her antidepressant medication. In fact, the only visits to me, as the months went by, were for the treatment of recurrent bronchitis brought on in large measure by a persistent and severe addiction to tobacco.

After several years in medical practice it is rare for anything new to surprise a family doctor. The description of Annie's smoking history, however, did test credulity.

"Doctor, you know when a youngster is seven or eight, and gets a few coppers, usually they wants to get candy with the money. I didn't. When I was seven or eight, I spent the bit o' money on cigarettes. An' I've been smoking ever since. An' I'm not going to stop."

How could she afford tobacco, living in poverty on the south coast with her unemployed brother and the only income a dole note?

"You could get a pack o' Target for 14 cents in them days. An' my brother used to chew Beaver, you know,

Doctor, that hard cake of tobacco that you cut off with a pocket knife and smoke in the pipe. He chewed it, most of the time, when he managed to get some. An' you know, when I was really hard up, he would take his chaw and dry it on the windowsill, and I'd smoke that."

There was no point in trying to get her to stop the habit.

"Doctor, I wakes up in the middle of the night to have a smoke. I've been doin' that for years. It's the only pleasure I got. I got no family; me cigarette and goin' to bingo is all I got to look forward to."

She knew full well the possible complications of smoking.

"Doctor, I wants you to promise me one thing. If I gets cancer, I don't want to have an operation. Just let me die in peace without havin' me chest cut open. They all dies any-way, operation or no operation, now don't they?"

Usually her recurrent bouts of bronchitis cleared up with routine measures — antibiotics, "puffers," and indoor rest for a week or so. But on one visit that took place about a year after I became her family doctor, the condition failed to clear, and she developed pneumonia.

Annie was persuaded, with significant difficulty, to enter the local hospital (under the care of a hospital-based physician), where the pneumonia improved. Unfortunately, a chest X-ray revealed a mass in the left lung.

She was encouraged to go to a hospital in St. John's so that a definite diagnosis of the nature of the mass could be made.

I learned about the events that occurred during that hospitalization in bits and pieces from reports from the hospital and, later, from Annie herself.

A biopsy was carried out on Annie during which a needle was inserted into the lung mass and a small core of tissue removed. The mass was cancerous. That night, a physician Annie had not previously seen came to her room and advised her of the diagnosis. He stated she needed further investigation including immediate scans of her liver and bones, with obvious need for treatment as soon as possible.

As usual, Annie was reluctant and said she needed time to think it over, whereupon the physician became "some rude": "Look woman, you haven't got any time to think it over. You've got six weeks to live." He stomped out of the room.

Next morning, Annie packed her little suitcase and walked out of the hospital.

Six weeks later, she appeared in my office and, between spasms of coughing, during which she spit up blood-tinged sputum into a tissue, she managed to tell me the details of her time in hospital. She was now quite ill, had lost considerable weight, and, on exam, demonstrated signs of advancing lung malignancy.

"Doctor, he told me I only had six weeks to live. The six weeks is up. What do I do now?"

Shortly before Annie's visit, I had received a full pathology report. It revealed that Annie was suffering from a particular type of lung cancer, a "small cell" cancer, which, in a certain percentage of cases, responds quite well to chemotherapy. In some cases the treatment even leads to complete cure.

Annie was so informed. She went home to think it over.

Two days later she returned; she would agree to go back to St. John's on condition that she would have no contact with the rude physician who had informed her of her imminent demise.

And so Annie did receive chemotherapy; a chest X-ray several months later revealed complete disappearance of the mass in her lung.

Several years later, I moved on to practice elsewhere.

When I left, Annie was still there, very much alive and well, still going to bingo, and still smoking her cigarettes, day and night.

NO BLAGARD *in* AUNT EMMA'S HOUSE

"I'LL BE HAVIN' NO BLAGARD in me house, do ye hear? I'm a decent woman an' if ye keep that up I'll be callin' down the priest, an' don't ye forget it!"

We teenagers of the pre-Confederation 1940s often went to Aunt Emma's house because in those days — before movies, TV, radio, and computers — our main source of entertainment was each other. Her little place was a rather nondescript affair, made up of a good-sized kitchen with settles lining the walls, a wood stove, which was lit winter and summer, and a table with a few locally made chairs. Free from the rigidity of school and our own homes, we wandered in and out, not particularly concerned about snow or mud on our boots. We almost always found members of our crowd in the place.

Aunt Emma was old — only God knows how old; to us, she appeared to be eternal. She was short, with a prominent dowager's hump that deformed her dress, usually a long dark garment that reached the floor, with an apron in front that she called a pinnie. She wore her grey hair in a bun on the back of her head, covered only when she went to church on Sundays and Holy Days. One eye was blind with a prominent cataract; the other eye, as far as we knew, was as good as new.

She spent her days in her rocking chair next to the stove, occasionally getting up to put in an assortment of fuel, or instructing us to do so. The main fuel was wood that she had obtained in a rather piecemeal fashion: Each winter day, the local men returning home from cutting firewood would have a starrigan on top of their load, which they threw over the fence into her garden. Come spring, Aunt Emma had a sizable pile of fuel for her stove. She supplemented this wood by burning peat from a bog nearby and, occasionally, even dried cow dung. She wasn't particular about what went into the stove as long as there was heat coming out.

Often Aunt Emma would spend the best part of the day asleep in her chair, rousing only when our laughter woke her. She would immediately assume, usually correctly, that an off-colour joke had been told and would berate us about the presumed blagard. She would then light her pipe and smoke for a few minutes before dozing off again, often dropping the pipe on the floor. Occasionally she would run out of the Beaver tobacco that she smoked and would take apart the butts from our cigarettes and use that, not being able to afford anything else.

She always maintained that, when she was smoking Beaver, her health improved, especially her chronically bad stomach. We teenagers paid very little attention to this affliction, considering that she was able to eat a daily meal of salt herring or salt cod cooked with several Jenny Lynn potatoes in a black bake-pot that was always in evidence on top of the stove. Her stomach complaints, whether real or imagined, were likely not helped by the fact that she was edentulous; she often spoke about this: "I can't chew me grub; all I can do is squat it."

She had a goat, which had arrived in the world at a neighbour's small farm several years before. It was the runt of the litter of three kids and the mother goat promptly rejected it. Aunt Emma was given the starving creature and, with some help from relatives and a concoction of Carnation milk, water, and cod liver oil (the first given to her by a local soft-hearted merchant, the last readily available), managed to keep the creature alive until it could feed on potato peels and the grass of early summer. The animal imprinted solidly on Aunt Emma, regarding her as its mother and, thinking itself human, would wander into the house whenever the door was open, often depositing goat buttons all over the floor. Aunt Emma would shout to one of us to "get that shagger out of here"; whereupon the goat would wander freely through the community, always returning, each day rewarding Aunt Emma with a small amount of milk and, every spring, two kids to supply some meat for the winter.

Besides the goat, Aunt Emma had a resident crow that had been rescued from a nest in a nearby grove of trees. The mother crow had been shot by a neighbour when it was found consuming his chicken feed. A nephew of Aunt Emma's rescued the crow, the only one still alive amongst three in the brood. He kept it alive by feeding it earthworms and bread soaked in water. After a week or so, he grew tired of the whole business and brought the creature to Aunt Emma, knowing full well that she would look after it. The crow, like the goat, decided that the world of humans had its positive aspects and determined to stay indoors as much as possible, rarely venturing outside her house. It became a source of amusement to all of us teenagers because the crow had learned to bow down with outspread wings whenever we entered the house, uttering a crow sound that we translated as "hello." The crow spent most of its time perched on a wooden clothesline above the woodbox, which it used as a roost, especially at night.

I don't remember Aunt Emma ever being seriously ill or needing hospitalization, though she was always complaining about some minor ailment or another. On one occasion, she did need the local doctor and called him in on a house call.

A granddaughter who had worked as a domestic with an American military family in St. John's had come home to visit after six months of employment. She had learned quite a lot during that short time — she had even developed a poor rendition of an American accent, to the point of saying NewFOUNDland, with emphasis on the middle syllable. As well, the young lady had stopped drinking the usual mealtime beverage — tea — and was now imbibing coffee, without milk or sugar, in the American fashion that she had observed amongst her well-to-do employers. On her visit back home she had brought a few pounds of ground coffee beans from her ample kitchen in St. John's. She encouraged all her relatives, including her grandmother, to try some. Aunt Emma reluctantly drank a cupful, mixed with goat's milk and a teaspoon or so of molasses.

Well, things went rapidly downhill from there. Within the hour, Aunt Emma developed severe stomach cramps, "looseness of the bowels," and, most worrisome of all, passage of blood "down through." The doctor was called; by this time she was shouting "that stuff is goin' to put me in the coffin!" and demanding the priest be called as well.

Both learned men eventually attended her and determined two things: she had the bleeding piles, and the Lord wasn't ready for her yet.

The prayers of the priest and/or the physician's ministrations worked: Aunt Emma recovered rapidly. Nevertheless, until the day she shook off this mortal coil, no manner of persuasion could convince her that the coffee had not been the cause of the problem.

Aunt Emma had many visitors besides us young people in the late years of her life. In that era, belief in the occult and the supernatural was common, especially amongst the illiterate. Aunt Emma was regularly asked for her predictions about the future fortunes or misfortunes of individuals in the community. Most of these people were young females. She would hold court with two or three of them while she foretold the path ahead, based upon the pattern of tea leaves in the bottom of the cup each one had just drunk from. If no definite pattern was evident, she would seek help from playing cards and, depending on the evolving configuration, predict (especially if spades or clubs) that the good lady would soon become involved with a "tall, dark stranger from overseas." As we all know, one did not need the help of the occult to predict this, since thousands of our young Newfoundland women found partners in American servicemen who were here at that time as part of the war effort.

On a more earthly level, Aunt Emma had a mysterious and widely recognized ability that confounded the medical people: a proficiency in curing warts. I observed the process in action. A small boy, his hands covered in warts, was told to go into the grass outside and bring in "four snails" (slugs). It was necessary that he do this on his own, without help from anybody. When he came back inside, she said, "Come 'ere, me little snot-nose, bring them things over 'ere." She took the four slugs, two to each hand, and rubbed the slime all over the warts. She then passed the slugs back to the boy and instructed him to "go over to the stove there, b'y, an' lift the damper and sling 'em in." When that was done, she announced that the warts would all drop off in two weeks. And, as often as not, they did.

Aunt Emma was a God-fearing individual and professed great faith. Every Sunday and feast day she attended church, attired in a special dress and an ancient hat, neither of which had changed for years. Just before Mass started, she was escorted up the centre aisle of the church, supported by two nieces who doted on her (especially when the congregation was watching), and then settled herself in the merchant-class area in the front pew. Although she said she went there so she could hear the whole ritual, she spent most of her time asleep, waking only when the priest was especially vociferous in shouting about hell's fire and damnation. She also woke up during the collection period if for no other reason than she wanted to be observed, wide awake, to never put anything into the collection plate. She felt that she had no reason to "buy her way" into heaven and, besides, what did you have to give when all that you received was a miserable $5 a month old-age pension? Such was the treatment of the elderly in pre-Confederation Newfoundland.

Aunt Emma died suddenly in her sleep one night in the summer of 1948. She never lived long enough to become a Canadian, but even if she had, her way of life would have changed little, with her wood stove, her pipe, her goat, her crow, and the teenage kids she welcomed daily into her home.

BESSIE, *the* FIGHTIN' TOM

THE PHONE RANG in the middle of a sunny Sunday afternoon in July. I was trying to make up my mind whether to go to my favourite pond to catch trout or lie around and enjoy a rare moment of peace and quiet. "Doctor!" the woman's voice said, without identifying herself. They rarely do. You soon learn to recognize everybody's voice anyway. "I got a problem," she said.

There you go, I said to myself. Peace and quiet. Hah.

"What's the trouble, ma'am?"

"The young maid is some upset."

Newfoundlanders often refer to their daughters as "maids" — a term out of the past — especially on the North Shore. I waited for further details.

"Bessie, it is. Got a hook in her mouth."

Bessie. Bessie? I had never heard of Bessie. I knew she had four daughters but that was a new name to me.

"Mrs. Halleran, who is this Bessie? I don't know anybody by that name in your family."

A visitor, maybe?

"No, no, no. It's the cat. Got a hook in her mouth. An' the young maid is some upset."

Invariably, back then, in the 1960s, all rural doctors were asked to look at animals occasionally. I didn't like doing it. God knows, I was busy enough looking after the problems of my human patients without tending to animals.

"Ma'am, I don't see animals. You know that."

"But, Doctor, it's the young maid's kitten, and she's got this trout hook down her throat and she's cryin' and bawlin' and I'm afraid she's goin' in the 'sterics."

"What?!"

"Rita. The young maid. Goin' in the 'sterics."

I do have a soft spot in my soul for suffering animals, inherited from my father, and she knew it. If it were up to me, I'd have the house filled with dogs and cats.

"Doctor, there's no vet this side of St. John's, and I can't afford to see one anyway. Doctor, you looked after Joey's cow when she got the milk fever ..."

"All right, all right, ma'am." No use arguing. "Bring her up."

"Now?"

"Now."

I mused as I waited, getting things ready. Can't let Rita go into the 'sterics. No sir.

I had a small collection of instruments for animals, mostly cast-offs from my practice, supplemented by a pair of wire-cutting pliers, a pair of gloves thick enough to protect my hands against bites, and a small sheet that could be wrapped around the animal for restraint.

By the time they arrived with the kitten, I had all these things ready, and was actually looking forward to the challenge.

Indeed, I did have a challenge ahead of me. My first look at that animal told me that. Bessie was a full-grown feline, lean of frame, mean of eye, with ears and face scarred from many past victorious conquests, and now ready to do battle with me.

"Mrs. Halleran, I expected you to bring a female kitten here. That's not a female, and it's not a kitten. That's a fightin' tom, if there ever was one."

"Yes, I knows that. But we thought she was a she when she was young. An' we still calls 'em she. But that don't make no difference. Do it, Doctor?"

No, I thought to myself, I suppose not.

"You goin' to put her to sleep, Doctor?"

"No." I'm not running a veterinary clinic here, lady, I said to myself. I make do with what I have.

All of the hooks I had removed previously were embedded in humans — usually in the hands or face. With judicious use of local anaesthetic, push the barbed end through the skin, then use the wire cutter. Nothing much to it.

But a co-operative hooked fisherman is one thing. A fightin' tom is another.

Now I instructed Mrs. Halleran on what lay ahead. I had a small table, narrow enough so that she could stand on one side, with her back up against the wall, restraining the animal, while I, gloves donned, worked on the other side.

The cat, sensing there was trouble ahead, hissed and snarled, with teeth laid bare and pupils wide with rage and fear.

We managed to get the small, narrow sheet around the tom, so that the torso of the body was restrained, with Mrs. Halleran holding the cat's legs and the head held firmly between her forearms, looking up at us.

Meanwhile, at the other end, the tail protruded from

the rolled sheet, flicking back and forth, harmlessly brushing my arms as I prepared for the ordeal ahead.

"Now, ma'am, you have to hold on tight." I could see the hook, far back in the throat, embedded deeply into the tongue. Going to be difficult.

I placed my gloved left thumb deep between the jaws to hold the mouth open to have a better look.

Oh, joy! The barb of the large hook had already worked its way back out through the mucosa of the tongue and was lying there waiting to be chopped off. A short distance away I could see the eye of the hook protruding, with a small piece of nylon twine still attached.

My plan was to grasp the barbed end of the hook with locking forceps, cut it off with the wire-cutting pliers, grasp the nylon twine and, bingo!, another reward in heaven.

Now imagine, if you can, the battle-scarred tom fighting the greatest of all his combats. Out of his throat came howls of rage, howls deep out of his primeval soul, out of his jungle ancestry.

I grasped the barbed end of the hook with the locking forceps.

And then, indeed, all hell broke loose.

Two things happened simultaneously. Mrs. Halleran, doing her job well, suddenly said, "Omygod, Doctor, I'm some weak." I looked up at a picture of facial pallour slowly sliding down the wall, letting go of her hold on the cat as she fainted away.

At the same time, I felt a strange sensation over my abdomen and legs, a warm feeling, warm and wet. The cat was now clawing himself loose, having dealt me the ultimate insult. Lord Jesus, I said to myself, why do I have to get myself mixed up in this business, at all? Why can't I stick to looking after snotty noses and bad backs? I stood there with my assistant on the floor and me with my hand attached to the forceps, the forceps attached to the hook, and the hook attached to the cat. But not for long. Well, sir, that had to be the fastest extraction of a hook in the history of the feline world. I did nothing. I merely held on to the forceps and the cat did the rest. In one split second, there was I holding the intact hook in the teeth of the forceps, pissed on, but victorious.

Mrs. Halleran recovered from her faint shortly and rose to her feet, apologizing profusely.

"I got a weak constitution," she offered, in explanation.

"Your cat certainly doesn't," I said, as she gathered up the beast and departed, full of praise for my surgical expertise.

HOOKED *on the* TRAWL

BACK IN THE 1970S, the vast majority of animals on the North Shore had a function and were very seldom kept simply as pets. Horses hauled firewood, plowed fields, and provided transportation. Cows gave milk, calves, and meat. Sheep provided wool, lambs, and mutton. I could go on, but let's pause for a discussion of canines, because this is a story about one of that species.

In the fall of the year, when the fishing season was all but over, the trawls were hauled in and the codfish cleared away. The trawls, some of them hundreds of fathoms long, with thousands of fish hooks attached, were thrown on the fields or onto rock walls before finally being sorted out and put away for the winter. During the fishing season, each time a trawl was pulled in, the fish that were considered vermin — sculpins, catfish, dogfish, etc. — were removed and thrown back into the ocean. On the final haul at the end of the season, these fish were often left on the hooks and thrown on the fields and rocks. Very quickly flies did what flies are supposed to do, and soon the rotting fish were being consumed by maggots.

Unfortunately, the smell sometimes attracted creatures other than flies.

Dogs on the North Shore then were usually hunting dogs — English setters, occasionally Irish setters, and beagles. I don't remember ever seeing one of these toy dogs now commonly kept as pets. Neither would dogs be kept as guard dogs — who would need them? Petty crime and break-ins were practically unheard of.

This is a tale about an English setter, your typical silver-haired hunting dog.

Early one Sunday morning, I was called by a woman from Long Beach. She was my patient and she owned an English setter, used by her sons to hunt partridge in the late summer and fall.

"Doctor," she said, "the dog came home this morning. He was gone for three days, and he's got a hook in his front paw. And, Doctor, his two hind legs is growed together!"

Now, God knows, as a family doctor in rural areas of Newfoundland, you never know what you are going to be confronted with next, what situations sometimes defy credulity. As well, along with the human workload, in emergencies patients occasionally ask for advice about their animals. And I had two setters myself. How could I refuse?

That morning, the woman having told me about her given-up-for-lost dog coming home with his hind legs "growed together," I thought, yes, there *is* something new under the sun.

"Now this, sir, is something I gotta see," I muttered into my tea and toast.

The lady, I remembered, had some vision problems and maybe, because of that, was seeing things not quite as they were, or should be.

"You're sure, what you're saying?" I asked.

"Oh, yes, Doctor, the two hind legs is growed right together."

Her relatives brought the dog into the outer waiting room of the clinic and the gentle creature — aren't all English setters gentle? — knowing help was at hand, lay on an old piece of carpet so I could examine him.

It was obvious what had occurred. The animal had been attracted to one of the trawls previously described and had one of his paws punctured by a fish hook — the typical, silver, three-and-a-half-inch-long barbed device commonly used on trawls. In trying to break clear he had been hooked again, this time in his hind paw, and in his efforts to kick at that had driven the barbed hook through and into the second hind paw. The silver hook was buried in the fur, of similar colour, and could hardly be seen.

The animal had been attached to the trawl for three days and had finally managed to chew off the lines ("seds") and hobble home on three legs.

The relatives were willing and able to restrain the animal if necessary, and I donned thick gloves to protect against a bite. None of that was needed.

The animal lay still while I injected local anaesthetic into the three paws, around the hooks. Two of the paws were already showing signs of infection. The barbs on the two hooks had been pushed through the flesh and were not buried in the tissue, so it was a fairly simple procedure to attach vice grips to each end of the hooks and, with a hacksaw, cut across the hard metal.

The whole procedure took about 10 minutes, and during all that time the animal raised not a murmur of protest.

When it was all over, he got up on his pain-free, hook-free legs and, wagging his tail, came over and licked my hand.

The main reward that a doctor receives is the gratitude

of his patients. That morning, when they offered to pay me, I refused to accept any money; I always refused, the few times I treated animals, back then, when all the world was young.

"Put some peroxide on the infected paws," I said, "and soak them in warm salted water for a couple of days, twice a day. And, before the season is over, bring me a brace of partridge. And tell whatshisname to get that bloody trawl off the rock wall. Next time, it'll be a damn cat and, man, I couldn't go through that again!"

NANA KNOWS BEST

"BUT NANA, I'M NOT SICK."

"Yes, you are, and Nana knows best. Now listen to the doctor."

Jimmy was a small boy, five and a half years old, brought to the clinic by his grandmother; he was her only grand-child and she, as expected, doted on him and worried excessively about his health.

"Doctor, he's some thin and puny, and right picky when he eats. There's hardly a bit of flesh on him, and I think there's something going on."

She had worked the best part of her life at the local hospital in various departments — the laundry, the kitchen, and as part of the cleaning staff. Along the way, she had come in contact with a tuberculosis patient and needed follow-up to make sure that she had not contracted the disease herself. Another time she was given prophylactic antibiotics for a period of 10 days after delivering food to the private room of a patient who was later diagnosed with meningitis. And now she had a daughter doing first-year nursing in St. John's, who, on her visits home, regaled her mother with wondrous tales of life in there.

For all these reasons she considered herself a cut above the average person in knowledge of matters medical and was not at all reticent in giving advice in this regard, whether requested or not.

The grandson had been born out of wedlock to her daughter, 16 years old at the time. The boyfriend was a year or so older. Some consideration was given to marriage, but not with any degree of enthusiasm since the grandmother-to-be looked upon him as a good-for-nothing. "Spends his time dodgin' around, with his hands in his pockets, doin' nothing. You know the type — here's me head, me ass is comin' — that sort o' fella." Shortly thereafter he took off for parts unknown, out west. A Christmas card arrived, once, with a $50 bill in it, and that was the last they heard of him. Or so she thought and, no doubt, hoped.

The daughter had gotten her life back in order; she finished high school and now was in nursing training. As often transpires in these situations, the grandmother took over rearing the little boy.

"Doctor, I want you to give him a good checkup. Maybe some blood tests too."

The examination revealed a bright, blue-eyed, fair-skinned little lad, with normal weight and height and healthy as a horse.

"You say he's picky about food? What did he eat this morning for breakfast?" I asked.

She thought before answering. "Oh," she said, remembering, "he had some milk, a boiled egg, and an orange."

Pretty good breakfast, I thought. Better than what I had.

"And what would you expect him to eat?"

"Doctor, I'd like him to have a bit of fried ham, or a nice bit of watered salt fish, like I haves in the morning."

Yes, and you with diabetes and high blood pressure, I thought to myself.

I assured her the exam was normal, that he was a healthy child, that no blood tests were needed, and to stop worrying.

But I knew that she would be bringing him in again, and yet again.

Sure enough, over the next couple of months she came to the clinic with the child on several occasions. Once she stated that Jimmy's "bowels were black," and she feared he was bleeding internally. It turned out the child had been picking blueberries the day before and, as we all know, small boys don't spend their time *picking* berries, they occupy their time eating them. Another time, she came in with a story that something had infected a neighbour next door. The patient, she said, had come down with fever, had been seen by really expert St. John's specialists, who had done all sorts of tests, none of which turned up anything.

The daughter in nursing school advised that this was probably an unknown virus of some kind and to keep a careful watch on her son, especially since the neighbour was back home, completely recovered. You can't be too careful, can you? Especially with a youngster, and he right puny.

Most of the visits, you see, were for trivial complaints, not worth wasting pen and paper discussing.

But for one.

Nana stated that the boy had been "shockin' sick" the day previous and had vomited on two occasions. During the course of the examination the boy mentioned (when he could get a word in edgewise, what with all the talk coming from the very concerned grandmother) something that he had not told his Nana.

"I eat a worm."

"You WHAT?" the grandmother screeched. "Sacred heart of Jesus!" She flopped into a chair, fanning herself with a sheet of paper that she grabbed off my desk.

"Hold on, now," I said. "Hold on a minute. You ate a worm?"

"Yes, but I didn't chew it up."

"Oh, holy mother of God, he's goin' to be the death of me!" She groaned and fanned herself more than before.

In all my years in practice, I had seen and looked after many children who had ingested many strange substances and objects. One child had been in the habit of feasting on gravel out in the front yard, without, it is noted, any disastrous result. Multiple times I had attended children who had swallowed coins, all of which had gone in one end, and, after a few days, out the other. But never had I come across a child eating worms.

"You want to tell me about that?"

"Joey told me that hens eats worms and that's how they makes eggs and worms is good for you. He says he eats 'em all the time."

"Joey?"

"Joey is his friend, Doctor, lives up the road. I told him to keep clear of him. Bad little bugger," she said, still fanning herself furiously.

"So you ate one?"

"Yes, but I didn't chew it."

"What then?"

"I trowed it up."

"You vomited it up?"

"Yes, with the pissgetti."

"Spaghetti. He had spaghetti for supper," she explained.

"You saw the worm when you threw up?"

"Yes, mixed in with the pissgetti."

Nana was finally able to get hold of herself. What if he hadn't vomited back the worm? What if it was a piece of spaghetti that he *thought* was a worm? Reassurance, once again, was the order of the day. Even if he had not gotten rid of the creature, no harm would be expected to occur to her darling boy.

Muttering to herself "My God, what next, I wonder," they took their exit, she whisking him ahead of her out into an uncertain and often cruel world.

∾

A couple of years passed. The daughter made frequent visits back home from school and continued to have a close relationship with her son. The boy loved his Nana but he knew full well who his mother was. On several occasions he accompanied her on weekends and short holidays, each time returning with exciting details of the excursions, related to the willing ear of his grandmother.

About six months after the daughter graduated, and now working at a hospital in St. John's, she came home for a weekend and dropped a bombshell into her mother's lap. Unknown to any member of the family, all the time she was in nursing school she had kept communicating with the boy's father in Alberta. She had kept this hidden from her mother because of the certain objections. The situation, however, now needed to come out into the open.

Jimmy's father had been working all these years, earning good money as a roughneck on a drilling rig, and had purchased a condominium in Edmonton. The young mother had been approached at a job fair in St. John's by a recruiter from Alberta and offered work at a hospital in the same city.

The grandmother knew what was coming next.

A couple of days later she came to my office, still in a state of emotional turmoil. She had not slept for a couple of nights and was tearful and exhausted.

But, as we all do when faced with the inevitable, she, after an initial period of hostility, was now accepting the facts. Her daughter and her grandchild would soon be 3,000 miles away.

"I'll be left alone now, Doctor, and that is something new to me. But I suppose it's all for the best. A boy needs a father and maybe he'll turn out to be a good one. He's got a good mother, and if things don't turn out, they can always come home."

Knowing how much she loved the two of them, especially the little boy, I knew that not only would the door of her house be open but so would the door to a very loving heart.

MARY

IT WAS IN THE 1940S, just after the war. Her man had gone away to Halifax, where he was to become a stevedore, a foreman on the docks. In order to get into Canada, which was then a foreign country, you had to have a normal chest X-ray in hand to prove that you didn't have consumption. The Canadians were leery of Newfoundlanders; they figured half them down there had consumption.

And here she was, all alone in Long Beach on the North Shore, with five children and her husband's elderly mother to look after.

Things were not good in rural Newfoundland in those days. Sure, if you lived in St. John's or Stephenville or Gander, and lived off the American bases, you could get by pretty well. But when the cod fishery failed that summer, her husband decided, along with a dozen others, to go up to Canada where, it was said, workers were needed and the pay was good — as long as they each had a normal chest X-ray and $100 cash to prove they were unlikely to become a drag on the Canadian welfare system. The $100, a princely sum in those days to the average rural fisherman, presented a problem, since none in the group had that amount of money. They solved that by pooling their funds, and as each one emerged from the immigration site, he passed the $100 to the next; in that way all of them were granted entry on a worker's permit.

He found the work he was looking for — and his wife remained in Long Beach, in a 100-year-old two-storey house with no central plumbing, a wood stove the only source of heat, and a stable filled with cattle.

And a house full of children.

The children's grandmother, God love her, helped out as best she could. But that winter, the daily running of the household from dawn to dark fell full weight upon the mother's shoulders: rising in the morning, lighting the stove, getting breakfast for the children before school, feeding the cows, sheep, horse, and chickens in the barn, clearing out the manure, pulling up water from the well with a bucket ...

I have listed only a small part of her chores. Let your imagination roam, and you will come up with a thousand tasks that I have not put words to. And she had to deal with them all.

One day, having returned from the root cellar with potatoes and turnips for dinner, she found her four-year-old daughter, Mary, complaining of abdominal cramps. Soon after that she developed severe diarrhea.

All over the island of Newfoundland that year, an epidemic of severe *Escherichia coli* gastroenteritis was raging through the population, mainly affecting the children. Many died. Health care in rural areas in these pre-Confederation days was often rudimentary. District doctors were poorly paid, poorly equipped, and came and went, often after only short periods of service to the community.

When Mary's condition worsened, and now she was having episodes of vomiting, as well as diarrhea, the mother brought her to a local hospital. The overworked attending doctor, on call day and night, 24 hours a day, complained to her about his workload and having to handle the crowd from the Western Bay district, as well as his own.

He examined the child, pronounced that the four-year-old needed a "good clean-out," and advised castor oil.

The mother, while most respectful of the mutterings of medical men, saw no sense in giving castor oil for a "clean-out" to a child who had had 12 episodes of diarrhea in the past 24 hours. In her wisdom and good common sense, she ignored the physician's advice.

Mary was now very ill. She was dehydrated, with sunken eyes and slack skin. She could hardly walk to the chamber pot. She constantly craved and cried out for water, which she would, almost immediately, vomit back up.

Ellen, a neighbour next door, heard about the child's illness and came to visit. The mother, at her wit's end with worry and exhaustion after four nights without sleep, broke down and wept, fearing the death of her little girl. Ellen tried to reassure her. But a child of Mary's age had died just the day before in a community close by; the mother's anxiety grew.

She could stand it no more. A telegram was sent to Halifax.

"Mary very ill. Want you to come home."

Three days later, he arrived by train.

In the meantime, Mary had been given medication which Ellen had brought over on the faint chance that it would help. It was called Paregoric, used then for various afflictions but rarely employed now. Almost immediately after receiving a small amount of the compound, Mary stopped vomiting, her diarrhea decreased in frequency, and her abdominal cramping ceased.

By the time the father arrived from the docks of Halifax, the child was up and around, drinking fluids, and asking for food.

He was overjoyed. He had feared a worse result, having read in a letter from home about the continuing epidemic on the island, and the children's deaths it had caused.

He stayed home for a week and then returned to Halifax.

That spring, he came home for good. Mary had recovered completely and had gained back all the weight she had lost during her illness.

With the money that he had earned in Halifax, he could outfit himself for the fishery with a better boat and better nets than those he had previously owned. That was the beginning of a long lucrative period in the commercial salmon fishery.

He came home from Halifax with a profound admiration for the Canadian way of life. On the shore a few years later, he became one of the main supporters of Confederation with Canada.

One night in 1949 we went to bed Newfoundlanders and woke up Canadians. In some segments of the population, there was sorrow and recriminations and bitterness at the loss of our independence. Some people wore black armbands, organized mock funerals, and swore they would never accept the Canadian old-age pensions and family allowances.

But ask the mother who had to endure a winter alone while her husband travelled to a foreign land to make a living — ask her what value that independence was and what good it was in rearing her children.

That morning in 1949, when she woke up, she was not just a Canadian; she was a very, very proud Canadian.

NORTHERN BAY: SEPTEMBER 9, 1775

There have been many descriptions in the literature of the great marine disaster of 1775. I feel my account to be unique in that I am a native son, having grown up beside, and fished in, Northern Bay (see map of the area on page 123). I listened to the oral tradition still rife within the population of the area; this story has long haunted residents.

IN EARLY SEPTEMBER 1775, a violent southeast gale struck the east and south coast of Newfoundland, so destructive in terms of loss of life and property that the storm has been listed as the seventh most severe to have occurred in the last 500 years. Upwards of 4,000 people lost their lives, most of them fishermen. Twenty per cent of the population of the French islands of Saint-Pierre et

Miquelon drowned. Most of the loss of life occurred on the fishing grounds offshore Newfoundland and on the coast of Newfoundland, mainly on the Avalon Peninsula and, most severely, in Conception Bay.

The storm has been referred to as a cyclone, with a storm surge of such height (up to 30 feet) that one writer mistakenly thought that it was a tidal wave resulting from an offshore earthquake. The hurricane likely caused more deaths in the northwestern North Atlantic than any other single disaster before or since.

As I grew up, there were occasional references to a long-ago marine disaster with great loss of life. There were also tales of screams being heard, screams like those of drowning men, whenever a southeast wind blew in the bay. It was said these sounds came from the "hollies," the ghosts of the men who had perished. My grandmother, Minnie O'Flaherty, could hear them on foggy nights when the wind was "in off the water."

Lewis Amadeus Anspach refers to that hurricane in his *History of Newfoundland*. Anspach, a clergyman, lived in Harbour Grace (as cleric and magistrate) from 1800 to 1812 and no doubt had first-hand details from people who were alive at the time of the disaster. He refers to ships in Carbonear and Harbour Grace being "driven from their anchors," but his comments are most pointed about the destruction that occurred on the North Shore. He writes of a cove "where upwards of 200 fishing boats perished, with all their crews." He does not name the cove, but oral tradition and subsequent writings identify it as Northern Bay.

According to local legend, there was one survivor: a cabin boy on one of the ships. He lived in the community afterward for an unknown period of time. He is still referred to as "the bedlamer boy," a bedlamer being a young seal.

All the other fishermen perished.

Then, as now, the dominant feature of the area is Northern Bay Sands, a crescent-shaped beach with the water to the north and south bordered by tall cliffs. The bay itself is small — less than a mile across, if we accept the boundaries as being Northern Bay Head to the north and Fox Point to the south.

Several features of the bay played a role in the events of that stormy night. The sand of the beach extends underwater and forms the bottom of most of the little bay. As well, while most of the area, especially to the north and south, is bordered by cliffs, the beach itself is not. To the west, beyond the beach, the land slopes gently upward and would have been covered by forest in 1775.

To the south of Northern Bay, from Fox Point to another rocky promontory called Salvage, are high cliffs for a mile or so, with no beaches in that area to speak of. The cliffs descend to the water's edge. That area is called, appropriately, the Highlands.

Although not a prominent feature, the configuration of the shoreline beyond Northern Bay to the north, and to a lesser degree to the south, forms a funnel with Northern Bay at the apex. This could cause a storm surge to be intensified under the influence of a violent southeast gale.

In 1775, the community of Northern Bay was sparsely inhabited by Irish and English descendants who lived off the land and the sea, mainly as small-boat fishermen. There was some agriculture, enough to subsist on, but the dominant feature of the landscape was forest.

Northern Bay offers good shelter from a northerly gale and excellent protection from a storm out of the southwest. During a southeast gale, however, Northern Bay is wide open to the North Atlantic.

In early September 1775, fishing boats had gathered in the waters of Northern Bay. A storm was brewing, and the small bay offered reasonable shelter in most cases. The boats were also there, in the meantime, to jig squid, which was used mainly as bait.

Many of the ships had come in from offshore fishing grounds, where they had fished cod all summer. The codfish, headed, gutted, split, and salted in the ships' holds, represented the summer's harvest from the greatest fishing area on Earth: the coastline and the Grand Banks of Newfoundland.

The ships were from several nations — British, Portuguese, Spanish, and some Newfoundland boats as well. The British ships were probably in the majority.

The ships from Europe, all heavily laden with fish, would be on their way home in the early fall. The plan would have been to ride out the coming storm, get some bait, fish a week or so on the Grand Banks, and then sail across the Atlantic to waiting families.

If Anspach's statement that "upwards of 200" boats were involved is correct, it would have made the waters of Northern Bay a very crowded place indeed.

The ships which arrived just before the storm struck would have anchored far out in the mouth of the bay. The rest of them would have anchored close to the middle section, avoiding close contact with the rocky shoreline and the beach and dropping their anchors in sand.

Local small-boat fishermen, knowing a storm was coming, would have left their boats anchored on the collars and rowed ashore in their dories, or, as I have seen in my childhood, hauled them high up on the beach in a small cove on the north side of Northern Bay. This area, situated in a break in the cliffs, is called "Isy Cove," a contraction of "Isaac's Cove." The distance from there to the squid-jigging grounds was no more than a few hundred yards.

I tell you this to assure you that the local inshore fishermen would be safely ashore, though their boats were certainly at risk. The fishermen who faced the peril of the oncoming raging southeaster were those who stayed on board their ships that night.

You can be sure the ships' captains and mates, knowing the signs of the impending hurricane, would have been watching anxiously as the wind speed grew, hoping that the southeast wind would veer into the north or into the southwest.

Unfortunately, it did not.

Realizing their predicament, some ships headed south for Salvage in an attempt to get outside that point and into Ochre Pit Cove or Western Bay. According to local lore, six of them made it. Whether they survived after that is unknown. Ochre Pit Cove and Western Bay are, like Northern Bay, wide open to a southeast gale. But unlike Northern Bay, they have a solid rocky bottom to which anchors could hold. The ships which didn't make it all the way around Salvage Point would have been driven ashore on the rocks to the north of Salvage, under the Highlands, with little chance of survival.

The ships left in Northern Bay felt the effects of the increasing storm. The wind howling in from the southeast would have been accompanied by the driving rain of a tropical hurricane. The wind increased in severity as darkness fell; the wave action sweeping in from Conception Bay increased in height, and the most dreaded and feared consequences began to occur. The heavily laden ships began to drag their anchors and drift toward the shore, some toward Fox Point, some toward the cliffs on the north side, but most in toward the beach. An anchor laid down into a sandy bottom would provide no protection in this situation other than slowing down the approach of inevitable disaster. During the night, some ships with lighter anchors — and more heavily laden with salt fish — drifted and collided with ships deeper in the bay. Driven by the incessant pounding of the waves, the ships tore each other apart.

Orders to abandon ship would surely be given, and some sailors would take their chances in dories or other small craft. I would expect some of these would survive in the water for a short period — it is difficult to swamp a properly built dory — and the men would attempt to row in toward the beach.

The chaos — the wind, the rain, the darkness (the only light from lanterns), ships colliding, and the inevitable violent contact with the rocky cliffs or grounding on the sandy bottom offshore from the beach — must have gone on for hours. The men had two choices: abandon ship or stay on board and hope for a miracle.

Meanwhile, the 30-foot storm surge would have swept all the small boats hauled up on the beach in Isaac's Cove out to sea. It would have rendered landing there, and on Northern Bay Sands, impossible. Anybody who is familiar with that area cannot but be astonished at the high waves that roll onto the sands during, and after, mediocre storms.

This one was anything but mediocre.

The storm surge had driven the ocean far inland, well up into the forested area beyond the sand. Thirty feet of storm surge is as devastating as a tsunami. It would have swept away all the stages in the fishing rooms on the north side of the bay as well as those on the south side near Fox Point. The homes of the local people high up on the cliffs on the north side would have been spared. The damage on Northern Bay Sands itself, since nobody used that area for their fishing activities, would have been confined to damage to the forest occasioned by the salt water rushing in and by debris being flung ashore from the destruction of the ships.

The scene that greeted locals at the break of day must have been beyond the most fertile imagination. The ships were either destroyed outright or pounded to pieces where they went aground. No sign of life was evident. Debris littered the shore all the way to Salvage: spars, masts, sails, and ships' timbers and planks all along the shoreline and up into the trees back of the beach. A massive amount of seaweed was thrown up on the sand, having been ripped off the sea bottom. Mixed in with the kelp were thousands of salt fish swept ashore after the ships had broken apart. Most horrifying of all were the bodies of sailors on the beach, among the trees, or floating in the water.

Later, as the locals searched the area for survivors, a terrified boy was found inland from the beach in a tree, where he had been flung by the storm surge.

When the storm abated, many bodies were recovered and buried in a mass grave near the beach. Over the next several months, bodies continued to wash ashore in Northern Bay and other communities in the area. The sea will give up her dead but will take her own time in doing so. Multiple burials were the responsibility of the local people. Local tradition has it that bones washed ashore on the sands of Northern Bay for years afterward.

The only communication with Europe in those days was by sailing across the North Atlantic, a sea voyage of several weeks. The families of the drowned fishermen learned of the disaster long after the event. Considering that often several family members would have been on a single ship, the impact of the misfortune on the relatives can only be imagined.

The sea, it is said, is made of women's tears. No doubt, in the fall of 1775, all over Newfoundland and in Europe as well, rivers of tears were shed.

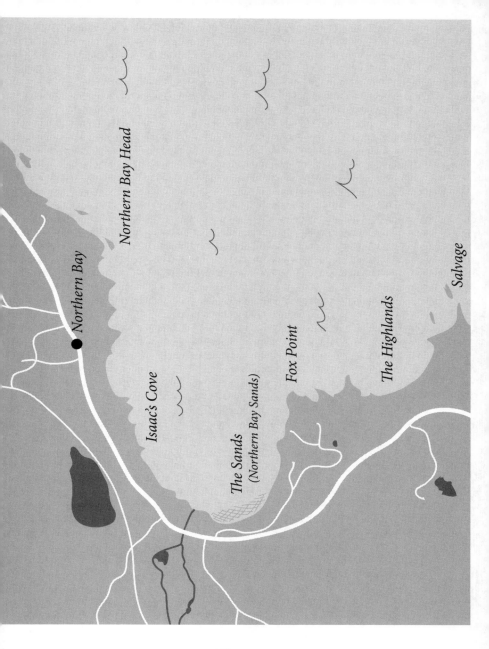

an HOUR BEFORE DAWN

IT WAS 3:00 A.M. when the phone rang. Three a.m., on a spring morning. An hour before dawn.

One ring was all that was needed. One ring and it was up to his ear. You learned that quickly on the North Shore. You didn't live next to the phone, but you certainly slept next to it.

"Doctor," she said, and named a name. "He just came up from the wake and he got a pain in his chest, and he wants you to come up."

She didn't need to identify herself. After years looking after their medical problems, and having grown up there, he knew everyone by their voice.

"Chest pain," he said, more to himself than to her.

"Yes. An' he's frightened to death."

Three days before, a woman had suddenly collapsed and died. She was in her early 30s, with no previous history of significant medical problems. She was a non-smoker, non-drinker, and ate a reasonably healthy diet with fish on the table three or four times a week, and salt intake kept to a minimum.

And suddenly she was gone. Without so much as a goodbye.

On the North Shore everybody knows everybody else. A priest on PEI once said that it is the God-given right of all Prince Edward Islanders to know the business of all other Prince Edward Islanders. And so it is on the North Shore of Conception Bay. Same thing.

The wake was held in the local funeral parlour. It went on for three days and three nights, 24 hours a day. The corpse was never left alone. Neighbours, friends, relatives were always present. Food was brought in because, of course, the living have to be fed. And drink too, a little nip here and there in the Irish fashion. Not too much, mind you, just a little sip to cheer up the sorrowing spirits.

The doctor was busy, more busy than usual those three days. The people, healthy and unhealthy, fearing the possibility of their own demise, flocked to his office with the mildest of symptoms, the slightest twinge of chest pain, the most trivial of digestive complaints. All were convinced that, like her, in the bloom of health, they were going down the same path. Not only was the doctor consulted, but the most worried and agitated availed themselves of the services of the priest and had requested the last rites.

Suffice it to say that none of these people, *none* of them, were anywhere near entry into the next world. Most chest symptoms were imaginary. The patients needed reassurance, and, in a few instances, a mild tranquilizer.

When the call came at 3:00 a.m., an hour before dawn on that spring morning, he ran through the medical records in his brain of the man who had spent the night at the wake and had just come home. In his 30s. No previous history of cardiac problems. No family history of such.

Same as the woman being waked.

He was about to tell the worried woman on the phone that he had seen 40 patients in the past few days, all with nothing wrong, all with chest pain, same as your man, and now please go back to bed and leave me alone. So I can get some sleep. But he knew it was useless to try and get back to sleep. He was never able to. There was always the nagging possibility of a disaster in the making. And, besides, the man she was phoning about was rarely in his office, not like some people, who are there, day after day, more for social interaction in the waiting room than anything else. The people you never see, you take notice of when called upon.

"Chances are there's not too much to worry about, but I'll come up and look him over."

He travelled up the shore a couple of miles and arrived 12 to 15 minutes after the phone call. She met him at the door.

She looked relieved.

"Oh," she said, "he's a lot better now, gone to sleep he is. I told him you were coming and he settled right down."

He wondered if he should disturb the sleeping man now that the problem appeared to be solved. But things are not always as they seem, and so he went into the small house — kitchen and two bedrooms and not much else — and saw the man on the bed covered up as if asleep.

He was stone dead.

That morning, as the dawn broke out of the northeast, he went from widow to relatives, and the man had many, to inform them of the sudden death. All of them, even in the turmoil of grief, had, with great good grace and in their own humble, rustic way, expressed gratitude for the doctor's part in the whole sorrowful episode.

Still, he had done nothing, other than to come when he was called, that night, an hour before dawn.

To this day he asks himself the same question, over and over: What if he had refused?

the TWO MABELS

SHE WAS NOT A WOMAN you would tangle with unless you were spoiling for a fight. Opinionated, rigid in her ideas of right and wrong, she was the undisputed head of her family and would continue to be so.

Mabel was tall, regal, with a prominent bosom and greying hair. When she came for her monthly checkup, she always wore a long, stylish (to her eyes) dress, and a hat that would be more appropriate at the horse races at Ascot than at a doctor's office in rural Newfoundland.

She suffered from "a touch of blood pressure," as she put it. For this she was given medication, which she took whenever she felt that her blood pressure was up, which she determined in a manner known only to herself. She ignored diet and weight control instructions. After all, she came from a generation in which weight loss was a sign of ill health and poverty, and, in extreme cases, consumption and sure death.

Her monthly appointment in the doctor's office was divided into two parts. In the first few minutes her blood pressure and weight were determined and advice given. After that, try as the doctor might, all discussion about medical matters was fruitless. She dominated the conversation from then on, berating whatever was irritating her at the moment. That generally included the merchants of St. John's, "millionaires all of them," she would say, rendering the "poor outport people" penniless. She voiced her disdain for the hatred that the merchants had for "the saviour of Newfoundland, Joey Smallwood" — hatred that was, she said, based on the fact that he was a bayman, and they were all filthy rich townies.

On other visits she would focus on situations closer to home. She got along with most of her neighbours, but not all of them, and she was merciless toward those unfortunates she regarded as straying from the straight and narrow. One particular individual was often a target of her barbs. "Every Saturday and Sunday he's on the beer," she would state. "Up he comes, up the road, staggerin' from one side to t'other, not knowin' whether he's comin' or goin', or on the way to the lunatic."

During these tirades, the doctor would try to get the conversation back to matters medical but would usually fail. After 15 minutes or so, she would pay her $2 visit fee and off she'd go for another month.

Besides herself, Mabel's family consisted of a husband and two children, the latter of course now adults, though she still referred to them as "the youngsters."

Her son was "gone away up to Canada" working in the tobacco fields "in a place called Tillsonburg." "Shockin' hot up there," she stated once, and he working with a bunch from the south who didn't mind the heat at all. She believed it was the last summer the youngster would go up there. Next year he'd be gone "down on the Labrador"; a body can stand only so much heat, you know.

Her daughter, a spinster, was in her late 40s and living at home. Her name was Mabel, same as her mother. Mabel junior and Mabel senior had accepted that spinsterhood was a permanent state of affairs for the daughter. "She could have got a man a dozen times," said mother Mabel, "but not a man would she let lay a hand on her." And, with a merry little laugh, added, "That's the only way to get a man."

Mabel's husband was a rather frail, ineffectual individual, weighing 50 pounds less than his wife and dominated by her in most aspects of his existence. He accepted his subservient position. He had had a shiny bald head since the age of 25. As if to compensate for the lack of hair on his head, he developed hair in excess everywhere else, with prominent bushy eyebrows and great mats of coal black hair on his body. He stated with some humour that he could, if he wanted to, comb his eyebrows back over his skull to cover his bald dome.

The family members, knowing their position and ruled by the matriarch, got along pretty well. The community regarded them as stable, God-fearing, and happy. They looked upon the community doctor as someone to call on in times of sickness, but recognized, as do most outport people, that life is unpredictable, and expected no miracles from the doctor, or anybody else.

One day the Mabels came in for a visit. Only one appointment had been made, but it was not unusual for two people to show up in the world of rural family medicine. Mabel senior had her "touch of blood pressure." Mabel junior was menopausal and, judging by her symptoms, having a difficult time. She complained of hot flashes, hot flushes, irritability, and moodiness. She had the full-blown syndrome.

"Doctor," the elder Mabel stated, "you got to do something. She's not fit to live with." She then went on with a long diatribe about what women used to do in the old days when they were on their "change." They often solved it, she said, by using herbs sent by relatives working as domestics "up in the Boston States," herbs that cured the flashes and, truth be known (hush, hush), rendered "matrimonial obligations" more enjoyable.

The physician prescribed hormone medication for the menopausal Mabel and a change of prescription for mother Mabel, giving her a more effective medication for blood pressure control. Next came the usual advice regarding weight control, avoidance of excess salt, avoidance of stress, and so on, all of which the doctor had no doubt Mabel senior would listen to with respect and then ignore completely.

One month passed. Both Mabels again came in to the clinic, this time with two appointments so the doctor could spend more time with them. Both were in tip-top shape. The younger one no longer had any of the symptoms of menopause. She felt like a teenage girl again, full of energy, and she had her eye on a certain man, which hadn't happened in years. Mabel senior was delighted with that development ("she'll maybe get him, God help us").

Meanwhile, Mabel senior was brimming with the joy of existence and happy with the world. Her blood pressure was lower than it had been in years. She had not a complaint about anything or anybody. All was sweetness and light.

The doctor was on the verge of congratulating himself on his superior clinical acumen and efforts to avail himself of the latest advances in the world of medicine, when he noted something was awry.

Somehow, along the way, the last month's prescriptions had gotten mixed up. For the past month, the older woman had been taking the hormones, the younger woman her mother's blood pressure pills.

Well, you can imagine the verbal consternation when the Mabels were informed about the mix-up and the obvious need to correct the problem. They objected to any change in the regimen they had followed for the past month, with the loudest complaints, naturally, coming from the mother.

He corrected the prescriptions, firmly labelling each as Mabel *Junior*, and Mabel *Senior*, and sent them off discontented and unhappy.

The doctor, up to the end of his period of practice on the shore, always had the suspicion that the two women continued to take the other's prescribed medication, and not her own. They denied it, of course, but still, deep down, his uneasiness was never quite relieved.

∿

The ultimate result of all the efforts of a physician in his practice is, sad to say, failure. As diligent as he may be, as expert in his knowledge and its applications as is humanly possible, someday all his patients will die. But that is not to say that, along the way, there are not great moments of triumph, satisfaction, and, often, hilarity.

Mabel had an abiding faith in what she called the Almighty. She spoke often of her faith to whomever would listen. This aspect of her life helped her overcome significant obstacles, especially in the days before Confederation with Canada, when there was widespread poverty amongst the scattered people of the rural communities.

On one visit to the doctor's office, she related what had occurred several nights before. It was her husband's birthday; to celebrate there was a cake and a few nips of rum. When you are 65, after all, celebrate all you want. You don't have too many birthdays left, as Mabel stated, in her wisdom.

She awoke in the middle of the night with "a shockin' pain in me belly."

"I had a bit of pig pork for supper, Doctor. I got that pain before, last year, after eating pig pork. I shouldn't be eatin' the damn stuff!"

Anyway, she woke her husband, and said to him, "Amos, go downstairs and bring me up that picture of the Blessed Virgin, you know the one, over there by the mantle, hangin' on the nail."

Down he went, half asleep, in the dark, and he with a bit of the drink still in him, and brought up the picture.

"Doctor," she said, "I put the picture on me stomach right where the pain was. Right there. First off, I didn't think it was goin' to work. But, you know, after a few minutes the pain started to ease off, and by the Lord Almighty, after another short while I dwalled off, and didn't wake up till dawn."

"An' you know, Doctor, I looked at that picture in the morning and damn it all, that wasn't a picture of the Blessed Virgin. That was a picture of Joey Smallwood!"

The doctor couldn't help but think that, amongst the considerable array of ammunition that medicine has to fight disease, relieve pain, and help the suffering of humanity, a new one had been revealed. Which just proves that you never knew what will come through that clinic door, or what unique individuals you will be called upon to deal with, day after day.

POOR UNFORTUNATE
ROOT CELLAR DWELLER

MY MOTHER, DURING HER LIFETIME, divided the people she knew into two groups: ordinary run-of-the-mill mortals like you and me; and the "poor unfortunates," by which she meant the downtrodden, living in circumstances inflicted on them by bad management, inferior genes, laziness, or plain bad luck. Bobby was of the latter category.

He was not one of my long-term patients. I knew him only a short time — several months at the most, long after he came to Newfoundland from Upalong. He could be quite talkative, however, and related many stories from the years before I met him.

Bobby had left Newfoundland some years before Confederation. He departed the North Shore to seek fame and fortune in Cape Breton when the coal mines were in full swing and where many Newfoundlanders had settled, some of them permanently. He worked in the mines for a while and did well financially until he developed emphysema — a severe lung condition brought on by exposure to coal dust and long use of tobacco.

When Bobby became disabled — so short of breath that he was unable to shovel coal anymore, making it impossible to earn a living wage — he went on the dole, up there on the outskirts of North Sydney. He had difficulty getting his dole allowance since he was not a Canadian but an alien from Newfoundland, but somehow he managed to convince a local "welfare officer" that he was related to the North Sydney O'Curtis family and indeed had been born and raised in Meat Cove, far up the north shore of Cape Breton. The welfare officer gave him the benefit of the doubt, and he lived for several years in a one-room shack on a vacant piece of land not far from North Sydney.

Although he was never comfortable about his health or finances, he did manage to get by, living from hand to mouth month by month on his dole handout. He had no friends in the surrounding communities — no wonder, since he was looked upon as an embarrassment. He visited the stores and church in threadbare clothes that he had worn years before in the mines, clothes now unfit for human use. His one-room shack had no indoor plumbing, as you might expect, and, as a consequence, people avoided him because of his appearance and his odour.

One day when he was visiting a local soup kitchen, he developed a severe pain in his back and down the left side of his abdomen, severe enough to cause vomiting and collapse. He was brought to the local hospital, where he was diagnosed and treated as having a kidney stone (renal colic). He passed the stone several days later and was discharged from the hospital, only to find that in his absence his shack had burned to the ground.

Without a home, and even more destitute than before, he was placed in an institution for the "disabled indigent," where he stayed for two weeks. When the administration checked into his background (more thoroughly than the welfare officer had), they discovered that Bobby was not a Canadian citizen, and therefore they had no hope of getting any payments for his stay in their care. He was given a one-way ticket by train and ferry to Newfoundland, and discharged. He attempted to cash in the ticket to buy food and get temporary quarters in a boarding house in North Sydney but was told the ticket had no cash value.

Penniless, unhappy, and homeless, he had no choice open to him other than to get on the ferry to Port aux

Basques and, next day, on the train across the island of Newfoundland to St. John's.

When Bobby arrived in St. John's, he was penniless, but he wasn't hungry. In those days the train ticket covered meals, and he had partaken liberally in the dining car, though people tended to avoid the table where he was sitting. A drunken lumberjack on his way home to Perry's Cove — after a three-month stint in Badger — had decided that Bobby was his "buddy," since his "woman had come from down the shore in a place called Spout Cove." He wasn't at all reluctant to sit with Bobby at the dining table for the long journey across the country. In fact, when they both checked into a boarding house on Brazil Square when the trip was finished, the lumberjack, Bobby's buddy, paid the $4 fee to cover the two of them for the night.

During the night, Bobby developed another attack of renal colic and needed admission to the old General Hospital. He was kept there until a full medical assessment determined that he had several problems besides his emphysema, including diabetes, high blood pressure, and, of course, recurrent renal colic. He was declared eligible for admission to the "poor house," the only institution available to house the indigent in St. John's at the time. That institution was, somewhat later, declared unfit for human habitation and shut down. Long before that happened Bobby gathered his few belongings and walked out, one month after being admitted there. He moved out to his roots on the North Shore.

Although his ancestors had immigrated to the area in the early 1800s and had lived off the land and the sea, they had all moved on — as had Bobby — to greener pastures. Bobby was the only one left to inherit a 5-acre plot of rural scrubland, now partly overgrown with alders. All that was left standing was a root cellar, kept up by a neighbour, who used it to store vegetables during the winter months. The old homestead had rotted into the ground.

When I first met Bobby and became his family doctor, he was living in his root cellar, and had been living there for several years.

A root cellar is basically a quadrangle of flat stones piled on top of each other to a height of 4 to 6 feet. Surrounding that is a thick layer of peat moss and clay, and surrounding that, a layer of rough stones and grass sods. The floor is always clay (earth). The roof is usually rough logs close together, covered by sods and clay. On top of the roof there is often a peaked triangular shingled wooden roof meant only to deflect rain outside the quadrangle of stones.

This is where people in rural communities store their vegetables in winter. If properly constructed, the interior is dark, damp, and never goes below freezing. Neither is it warm. But as many early settlers in eastern Canada know, you don't freeze to death in a root cellar. You can survive in there when you have no other choice.

Bobby had constructed a rough wooden shack at the entrance to the root cellar. In there he had a wood stove with a stovepipe, a table, and a few wooden chairs. He spent most of his time there, retreating and sleeping in the root cellar section of his abode during cold nights in the winter.

When I examined Bobby for the first time, he was unkempt and almost blind. His diabetes was poorly controlled, with blood sugars in a range ordinarily requiring hospitalization. He needed frequent injections of insulin to control his blood sugar, ideally administered every six hours. He refused hospital entry, and arrangements were made for a public health nurse to visit to teach him how to administer insulin on his own. Meanwhile, I agreed to visit him daily.

It soon became apparent that frequent insulin injections were, under the circumstances, beyond all range of common sense. He was placed on oral anti-diabetic medication that needed to be given once per day. Under this setup he appeared to be improving slightly.

I saw Bobby frequently in the months following my first introduction to this "poor unfortunate." He was not a bitter man. He accepted his lot in life, harbouring no animosity about his treatment "up there in Canada." I spoke to him about that, especially about his little shack getting burned while he was in hospital with renal colic. He laid no blame, cursed no fates, held no grudges.

One morning, on my daily visit, the small stooped blind man did not greet me at the door of his place. I went in, fearful — and found him, on the floor, dead, dead for many hours before I had arrived.

And so passed on one poor unfortunate. Life was not easy on him — but he did his part, nevertheless, shovelling hundreds of tons of coal that, possibly, warmed your relatives and mine and turned the wheels of industry.

There, but for the grace of God, go I.

DEATH *on the* HIGH SEAS

"THERE'S A BOAT COMING IN with a dead man on board. Fishing boat. Arriving around noon."

I was on call that weekend in the early 1960s, one of a group of physicians designated as "port doctors" in St. John's. Back then, the coastline of Newfoundland was swarming with foreign fishing ships taking advantage of the 12-mile territorial limit, which would be extended, soon afterwards to 200 miles. Most of these ships were Spanish or Portuguese — people with a tradition, dating back to the time of Columbus, of crossing the Atlantic in their sailing vessels, spending the summer and early fall on the Grand Banks, and then sailing back home with their holds laden with tons of salt codfish, back to the Iberian Peninsula for the winter.

These short, muscular, swarthy fishermen were a

common sight on the streets of St. John's. Their boats came ashore for a variety of reasons: to ride out a hurricane, to bring in a sick shipmate, to shop for gifts for relatives back home, and, often, to buy the lightly salted codfish cured on the flakes of the fishermen of eastern Newfoundland — a delicacy for them, fit for celebrations during the Christmas season and other feast days.

Theirs was not an easy life. I have been on board the ships. The fishermen lived in cramped quarters from spring until fall, often subsisting on daily meals of fish and more fish, enduring long hours of work from dawn until nightfall, especially when the fish were plentiful. Sometimes when the codfish moved offshore or up to the northern waters, the boats ranged as far away as the coast of Labrador and even to southern Greenland. Under these circumstances, the fishermen, usually exposed to the warm foggy waters of the Gulf Stream on the Grand Banks, would have to contend with the ice and cold of the Labrador Current. The ordinary seamen, the ones taking the fish out of the nets or off the trawls, would be subjected to extreme cold for long hours at a time. I have seen them brought in to St. John's with gangrenous fingers blackened from frostbite, fingers beyond all hope of therapy, and eventually needing amputation. These men, who depended on a healthy functional pair of hands for their future livelihood, would often be doomed to an uncertain and difficult future. Certainly they were of no further use in the fishing boat.

That morning, when I received the call from the secretary about the boat arriving with the deceased man, I proceeded down to the docks long before noon to await the ship. I loved the smell of the salt water, the hustle and bustle on the wharves, with sailors milling around speaking languages from God-knows-where, and local fishermen selling cod fillets, tongues, and other edible parts of fish caught that morning. I sat in the car next to a Portuguese fishing boat and watched as the men threw bread soaked in wine onto the wharf to be gobbled up by the pigeons. These creatures, soon inebriated, were grabbed by the Portuguese fishermen. When you've eaten nothing but fish and hard tack for three months, pigeon stew is a feast.

Soon the boat with the dead man arrived and docked portside, close by my vehicle, flags at half-mast. I walked to the gangway, black bag in hand — enough to identify myself as the port doctor of the day.

I met the captain and spoke with him through an interpreter supplied by the port authority. During the interview he was agitated, constantly pacing the cabin, distressed at having had to come ashore when the area where he was fishing was yielding great hauls of prime codfish. He wanted to get all this business over with and get back, as soon as possible, to the fishing grounds.

According to the captain, the man had died of a heart attack. He had suffered upper abdominal and low chest pain for three days, sudden in onset and accompanied by sweating. The first-aid man on board felt it was simply an attack of indigestion and various stomach remedies were administered. However, symptoms persisted until eventually the patient became comatose and then expired. It was obvious to the captain that the only explanation for the whole unfortunate affair was that the man had died of a "bad heart."

The dead man had two brothers on board, who had caused problems by insisting that the patient be brought to shore several days before his death. The captain had refused to do so because of the advice of the first-aid man — but also because of the disruption it would cause to the lucrative fishing going on at the time.

I examined the body: a young man, 25, muscular, with no signs of jaundice, emaciation, injury, or other obvious cause of death.

I was asked to sign the death certificate stating that he had died of a heart problem. By doing so, the body would have been removed from the ship, flown back to his home country, and the captain and crew would have rapidly gone back to the fishing grounds.

I refused. Young men of 25 years don't expire from a heart attack. They die of a multitude of problems but rarely from a heart attack. I refused to sign the death certificate. I requested an autopsy be done as soon as possible. The captain, now more upset than before, kept repeating a word that the interpreter stated was the Spanish equivalent of "bullshit."

The autopsy revealed that the young man had died of a perforated ulcer. In this condition, an ulcer erodes an opening through the wall of the stomach, which then discharges acid and gastric contents out into the abdominal cavity, leading to general peritonitis. A horribly painful death follows within 24 to 36 hours.

If he had been brought ashore sooner, he could have had surgery to repair the problem and, possibly, his life saved.

The brothers and many members of the crew, on learning of the autopsy findings, refused to return to the ship and had to be flown home to Europe.

The ship, with a skeleton crew, sailed back across the Atlantic with the hold half empty.

a DIFFICULT PATIENT

HAROLD LOOKED AT ME with a grin on his face, the usual expression he wore whenever he entered the office.

"I'm a sick man. I'm not well."

He always waited to see how I would react to that statement. Waited a few seconds ...

"I'm almost gone."

He didn't look ill. He never did. He enjoyed the shock effect, the same tactic he employed with the staff in the front office when he came in without an appointment. He rarely, if ever, made an appointment.

Harold was 60 years along, overweight, and diabetic. Often he came to the office with the smell of alcohol on his breath.

"You look OK to me," I said. "Not like you're on the way to the graveyard."

I knew him of old. The entrance that morning was the same as before, repeated many times through the years.

"Check me over. You'll see how sick I am. Damn nurse out there wasn't going to let me in. No sir."

Blood pressure cuff on his arm. Up some, nothing to worry about.

"Make an appointment next time. Jumping ahead of everyone, that's what you're doing."

"That crowd out there — not a one of them sick — out there gabbin' and talkin' and goin' on. Especially the women. Out there 'cause they got nothin' better to do. And here I am kept waitin', and I a sick man."

Blood pressure repeat, five minutes after first reading. Down now. Heart sounds OK. Lungs clear. No swelling of the ankles. Weight, 3 pounds over his last weigh-in, two weeks ago.

"What was your breakfast this morning?"

"Two slices of baloney and a pork chop."

"A pork chop?"

"Yeah. Left over from last night. I didn't want the cat to get at it."

"Piss-poor breakfast for a diabetic, I'd say."

"Right, Doc. But I got to keep goin'. Out on the river every day, most days, guidin'. Just like me father."

Blood work, out of his finger. Sugar level 16; too high. Way too high. I tell him.

"I know," he says. "Up on bust. But it's not fasting. Down if I was fasting."

Right on. He knows what is right and what is wrong, does Harold.

"When did you last have a drink?" I ask.

"Two weeks ago."

Lyin' eyes, looking at me.

"Booze is going to kill you, Harold."

He stared at me. Thought a few seconds. Sizing me up.

"It didn't kill me father. Lived to be 86. Out on the river from April till October. Guidin' the sports. The best guide ever from Renous River. Went into the water once, in the spring, with the ice runnin'. Up there at the mouth of Cains. Floated in the early dawn all the way down, all the way down, with his waders half full of air, to Doctor's Island, where the water got shoal. Walked ashore he did, an' he half-froze to death, almost.

"You know what kept him alive?"

He looked at me, knowing that I was curious about how his father had survived, floating miles down frigid water that had drowned the sport fisherman he was guiding. Yes, I knew parts of the story from previous tellings.

"Rum," he said.

"Rum?"

"Yes. Every time he went on the river, guidin', he kept a mickey of rum in his vest — sometimes he kept two mickies in there — and when he was floating down toward Doctor's Island, with pieces of ice all around, downstream, he took a swig now and then, enough to keep him alive; that and a prayer, now and then, to the Almighty. When he walked ashore on Doctor's Island, he forgot all about the Almighty and finished off the second mickey all in one big gulp, enough to warm him up and live on another five years.

"He lived well into his 80s and that's what kept him goin'. Rum didn't kill him; it kept him alive well beyond his three score and ten."

Harold gazed at me with that look of success. There are times when you have to look success in the face. Booze is bad. Tobacco is bad. Overeating is bad. But sometimes good genes trump all else.

"You know what Winston Churchill had for his breakfast in the morning? I'll tell you. A glass of raw rum. And a cigar. Every morning. And you know what? He won the war. Beat the bejesus out of Hitler."

I didn't bother telling Harold that Churchill imbibed only good Scotch whisky and never, ever, drank gut-rot black rum; if I had, he would have come back with an answer to put me in my place.

That was Harold — still there when I moved away, still on the river guidin', still living life to the fullest.

the OLD LADY *with the* BREEDING CATS

I ALWAYS ENJOYED HOUSE CALLS. I would say, without statistics to the contrary, that in my 40-plus years in family practice, I have made as many, or more, house visits as any other doctor in Canada.

My old chief of medicine used to say that you never got to know your patients until you visited them at home. A neat house, where you could eat off the floor, he'd say, was one thing. Having to crawl over beer bottles and boots in the porch is another.

I had visited many homes in St. John's before starting practice on the Conception Bay North Shore. I'd been into the homes of the very poor where I have seen the bathtub filled with coal and the children sitting down to a lunch of a can of tomatoes. The vast majority were not like that, of course, but some were similar, or worse.

The conditions I found on my first house call on the shore, however, were not what I was expecting. I had grown up in the area and was acquainted with the circumstances of the average family.

On my first day in practice — indeed, during my first morning in office — the village postmaster came in to prepare me for the situation I was about to confront.

He related details of the misfortunes of an elderly lady whose husband had died about two years before my arrival. Prior to his death, the couple had requested that the Department of Welfare supply a caretaker to help out with their daily needs. They both were in their mid-70s, living in a dilapidated two-storey house which, on inspection, was declared unfit for human habitation.

The department social workers recommended that the couple be placed in a senior citizens complex in St. John's. The couple refused; they had never been to the city — the farthest they had travelled out of Angashore Bight was to Carbonear, 20 miles up the shore; and their two cats would not be allowed to accompany them.

The ancient homestead was beyond any hope of reasonable repair. The roof was sagging and leaked every time it rained. The only source of heat was a wood stove vented by a chimney that was falling to pieces and declared a fire hazard. Toilet facilities were chamber pots and an outhouse, at times inaccessible in the winter. The only source of light was two kerosene lamps — again, a fire hazard. They had no electricity.

Considering the feelings of the aged couple and the fact that facilities for the long-term institutional care of the elderly were in short supply, the government department decided to build a small dwelling close by the old homestead. The new home would supply the basic needs of the couple for the rest of their lives. The old place would be demolished.

The finances made sense. The land on which the proposed building was to be built was supplied free of charge; the couple had owned it dating back beyond the memory of most people in the community. Unemployment in the area was rampant and capable carpenters, plumbers, and electricians were looking for jobs. Finding workers to build the new place would not be a problem.

The small dwelling, measuring approximately 20 feet by 20 feet, would contain one bedroom, a bathroom, a common living room-kitchen, indoor plumbing, and an oil stove.

The plan was to move the couple into the new abode in mid-December so they could enjoy Christmas for the first time in their lives without having to contend with a wood stove and trips outside to an outhouse.

In late November, as often happens in eastern Newfoundland, a severe winter storm struck the area, with heavy snow followed by unusual frost. The neighbours, having dealt with the problems inflicted on their own homes by the storm, eventually got around to visiting the two old people. They found the man dead in his bed, dead for several days. His wife had kept the wood stove going, having determined, in her senile state, he wasn't dead but merely frozen stiff. Her means of trying to revive him was to place several heated beach rocks enclosed in towels or knitted woollen stockings next to his body.

After the funeral, the widow, with her two cats, moved into the new place. The government arranged for a caretaker to spend six hours a day caring for her needs, getting her groceries, and cooking her meals. This arrangement worked out well for the first few months. After that, the hired workers would last several days — then quit.

When I arrived on the scene, the postmaster told me in no uncertain terms that it was my responsibility to do "something" with that unfortunate woman.

That afternoon, when I did a house call to the small home, I realized why "something" had to be done.

I opened the door of the small cottage, black bag in hand, my first house call on the shore. What struck me first was the smell — an overpowering stench of cat feces and urine, combined with a wave of heat coming out the door — and then the sight of multiple cats, small and large, scurrying across the floor as I entered.

I went in. Ahead of me was a room with an oil stove, a table and two chairs, and a door to the right leading to a bathroom. Over to the left was a door, partly ajar, leading into the bedroom, into which I had seen the cats disappear.

The old lady had been told that the new doctor was coming to give her a checkup. When I opened the door to her bedroom, the look she gave me was not one of surprise or hostility but probably the same tolerant look she gave to the various social workers who occasionally invaded her domain.

She was lying in bed, fully clothed, and partly covered by filthy bedsheets, blankets, and old coats. In amongst the bedclothes was a hodgepodge of mouldy bread, biscuits, and pieces of bologna gone green around the edges.

Meanwhile, the cats had disappeared under the bed. I had been told about this by the postmaster. The only place the cats felt safe was under her bed and it was there that they went whenever a stranger — basically anybody but the old woman — entered the house. The cats were never allowed outside.

When the husband was alive, the female cat — one of the two that they had kept for several years — regularly produced a litter of kittens. He prevented this progeny from reproducing by the common practice on the shore of placing the small animals in a burlap bag with a rock and throwing the unfortunate creatures over the wharf. She always objected to this method of treating "God's innocent creatures." Now that he was gone, she got her wish. The cats were allowed to breed without restriction — and breed they did. On that first house call, I counted 28 cats, using the space under her bed as their hiding place and toilet. There were areas in there where cat feces was 6 inches deep.

I examined her and found nothing physically wrong, other than the usual issues of aging — after all, she was 79 years old. Mentally she was senile, with her cognitive powers impaired. She was not on any medication; a physician had not visited for several years. The last time she had been seen by a doctor, she related to me, she had had "trouble with the womb," which she cured with a boiled mixture of onions and rhubarb.

Over the next several days, I spoke to the various people who had taken some responsibility for her care —

her clergyman, the postmaster (a kind-hearted man who was recognized as a leader in the community), and the social worker, who had just taken over her care and was not yet fully appraised of the ongoing situation.

The clergyman was especially helpful. He was the person who paid her account at the grocer, her electricity and oil bills, and cashed her old-age pension allowance when she marked her X — she was illiterate — next to her name handwritten on the back of the cheque. He attempted, along with his wife, to try to get rid of the cats that had taken over her house.

She refused any restrictions on these animals and wanted the oil stove turned up on high, even on hot days in the summer, to keep the cats warm. The gauge on the oil stove was never turned down.

To remove a person forcibly from his or her residence and normal way of life requires evidence that the person has committed a crime, is a danger to himself, herself, or others, or a danger to property. Mrs. —— could not be removed from her residence based upon any of these legal requirements. Six months before I arrived, the Department of Welfare had tried a different tactic. A geriatric nurse examined the old lady to determine if she could be declared a "neglected adult." If she were so declared, then she could be taken without her consent and confined to a nursing home.

It did not work. The application was turned down. Although the elderly lady was certainly suffering from a degree of senility, she was not physically disabled or suffering from any significant physical illness.

I tried, along with earnest pleas from her clergyman and his wife, to persuade her to move away from Angashore Bight, without success. She stated in terms that would brook no argument: "I'm not leavin' me cats."

Six months after I arrived, in the late fall, with the cold weather coming on, I noted that the lady appeared particularly frail but without any overt signs of impending physical calamity. She looked pale and had lost her appetite. She was losing weight. Her grocer continued to deliver, as per her orders, meat, fish, sausages, bologna, and other supplies to her home. The question was, of course, how much of that food was ingested by my patient and how much fed her cats.

In the late fall I did blood work on her at home and found that her hemoglobin was 6, well below normal. I convinced her, again with considerable support from her clergyman, to agree to go to the local hospital for a three-day visit for investigation of her anemia. Some tests were carried out. Others were recommended but were too invasive, in her opinion, and she refused.

Her home had been left with enough food and water for the three-day absence to sustain the cat multitude. The clergyman visited the place on the morning that she was to be discharged and discovered a major disaster. The flame in the oil stove had gone out and the place had been left in freezing temperatures. The water pipes had burst, as had the flush box, resulting in flooding all over the floor — now a sheet of ice. Most of the cats were dead, including a litter of six kittens.

Once again, the old lady had no home fit to live in. Major renovations were necessary, entailing considerable costs, and ideally deferred until the spring.

The social workers at the hospital swung into action. They now had a patient with a significant degree of senility and an untreated physical problem, undiagnosed as to cause.

She was declared a "neglected adult" and transferred to a nursing home in St. John's.

I never saw the lady again. Six months after being transferred to St. John's she died of metastases from cancer of the bowel, the cause of her anemia in the first place.

She was buried in Angashore Bight.

LAWRENCE'S HAVEN *of* PEACE

IT DIDN'T TAKE LONG for Lawrence to realize he had made a mistake, after moving to the North Shore from Bonavista Bay: He should have stayed where he was.

Old men dream dreams and make foolish decisions sometimes, thinking that the happy past can be repeated into the future. Lawrence was three score and ten when he packed up bag and baggage and moved in with the Widow Mulcahey over on the shore of Conception Bay North. He had never visited that area before, other than once as a boy when his father had caught a massive haul of salmon in his cod trap and had gone door to door for several days selling the salmon for five cents a pound. To Lawrence, moving over there was like going into a foreign land.

Lawrence was a widower. His wife had died, child-less, years before, leaving him to subsist on an old-age pension in a barebones two-storey outport house. When the cod moratorium of the 1990s decimated the fishery in his small community, most of the young people moved away, leaving behind only the elderly and the chronically unemployed. With no caring relatives in the area, Lawrence realized he would soon have to move away from the place where he had spent his life, possibly into a distant nursing home.

I became his family doctor soon after his move to Conception Bay. He spoke to me at length about how a clergyman from the shore, saving souls in Bonavista Bay, had acquainted him with a widow in Mackerel Gut, who was living, as he was, childless and alone. Knowing that a wood stove can boil Jiggs' dinner for two as cheaply as for one and a bed is warmer in the winter with two under the blankets, he decided, after discussions with the Widow Mulcahey, to make his move. He sold his house in Bonavista Bay for a nominal sum — real estate values had been decimated along with the cod fishery — and moved to Mackerel Gut.

A wedding was held, with the usual fanfare and well wishes all around. At the ceremony, the preacher spoke at length of Christian fellowship and a long happy life in the future. Afterwards, at the wedding celebration, one old codger, himself living alone, said to Lawrence: "My son, you got 'er knocked — two old-age pensions coming in — b'y, I wish I had got ahead o' ya, but she wouldn't have me. She's too particular."

The small amount of money that he had received for the sale of his home in Bonavista Bay was paid out to a contractor, who added an extension containing indoor plumbing to Mrs. Mulcahey's home. A year or so later, when he felt free to talk to me, knowing that what he said was kept in strict confidence, Lawrence said the only bene-fit that he received from his move was that he now had a toilet, bathtub, and running water.

The initial warm welcome in Mackerel Gut gradually cooled and, little by little, he began to feel like an intruder in the home. Mrs. Mulcahey had lived alone for years after her husband died, except for rare visits from a distant rela-tive. She now had to cope with a man in the house disturb-ing her routine, invading her bed, stomping snow in her porch, and expecting to be fed. In many subtle ways, with-out saying so outright, she made him feel that he was an irritant to her accustomed way of life.

He was quickly banished from her bed with complaints

that she couldn't tolerate "the old man smell." From then on he slept in a small storage room on the northwest side of the house that had never been used as a bedroom because it was so cold in the winter months.

I attended Lawrence many times down through the years that he resided in Mackerel Gut. Office visits were the most pleasant because we could talk in complete privacy — house calls were another matter altogether. She was always in attendance, constantly interrupting and talking over him, correcting and belittling him whenever he managed to get a word in. I saw him reduced to embarrassed tears because of her treatment of him in my presence. Finally, all requests for house calls ceased. I saw him, after that, only in the office.

He confided to me that her disdainful treatment of him occurred whenever people visited the home. She appeared to relish criticizing him in front of visiting neighbours, often relating embarrassing personal incidents.

Close by the residence, *her* residence (as she so frequently stated), was a small barn in which the couple stabled a cow and calf, purchased soon after his arrival on the shore. In the winter months, Lawrence took pleasure in looking after two creatures that needed his attendance and depended on him for their care. Next to the barn was a small storehouse; Lawrence renovated it, installed a wood stove, an old sofa, and a few chairs, and over the door a sign: "HAVEN OF PEACE."

I visited Lawrence in his haven several times. Often, when I arrived, unannounced, I would find the men of the community sitting next to the stove, most of them smoking pipes or chewing tobacco, spitting into the fire, and talking about the best way to grow round blue potatoes or Formanova beets or early cabbage. Initially my presence put a damper on the goings-on, but after a while, when they realized that I could talk their language, and could grow vegetables just as well as they could, I became part of the group in Lawrence's haven.

I knew that he now spent most of his waking time in the barn and in his haven, at ease with his animals and the men of the community. Without that ongoing respite from the stress of living with his wife, he would have become depressed and despondent. On one occasion he told me that he was considering applying for entrance into a nursing home up the shore a ways in Carbonear or Clarke's Beach. "The happiest time I am, Doc, is when I'm in the barn, in the dark, sittin' on an upturned bucket smokin' my pipe and listening to the cows chewin'."

One morning, in the dead of winter, Lawrence awoke and went downstairs to light the wood stove and cook breakfast. He was puzzled that his wife did not appear as soon as the kitchen had warmed up, as was her usual routine. Not wanting to disturb her sleep, he went out to the barn to feed the animals. When he returned, she had not yet made her appearance. He waited a few minutes and then went to her bedroom. She was in bed, trying unsuccessfully to speak, unable to move. She was hemiplegic, paralyzed on one side of her body, having suffered a massive stroke during the night. Lawrence had no concept of the diagnosis or the seriousness of her condition; he only knew that she needed help.

The ambulance transported her to the local hospital. Weeks of therapy and the best of medical care failed to improve her severe disability. She would never walk or speak coherently again.

The social service people, on advice of medical personnel, and knowing that her elderly husband could not care for her, placed her in a nursing home for ongoing care. Soon afterward, she was transferred to a level-three institution in St. John's.

She never returned to Mackerel Gut.

Lawrence lived on for many years, getting along well with the local people in his adopted community. He took great pleasure in inviting them into the house whenever possible, where they smoked their pipes, told stories of days gone by, and talked about growing Aran Blue potatoes, alfalfa hay for the cows, the price of salt herring come the fall of the year ...

WILD RIDE *to* CARBONEAR

WHENEVER I HEAR ABOUT a pregnant woman wanting to deliver her baby in her home rather than in a hospital, I cannot but be reminded of a woman I met many years ago when I was a young doctor just out of medical school. I was doing my internship, treating, along with my colleagues, the halt and the lame and the blind from all over Newfoundland pouring into the old General Hospital in St. John's. The woman was 50 years of age, or thereabouts, and had come into the hospital for the removal of a lump in her breast.

Before surgery, as was the usual routine, she was examined and asked details of her medical history, family history of illness, obstetrical history, and so on. Everything was fairly straightforward, except for her description and consequences of the birth of her one and only child.

She was 18 at the time, a strong healthy girl, married and living on the coast of Labrador during the depression of the 1930s. When the time came to deliver her baby, the local "midwife" — a well-intentioned granny who had assisted at births many times previously — was called. Labour pains ensued and, just eight hours later, the rapid delivery of a 10-pound healthy baby.

She survived with a serious problem, which she tearfully described: "Doctor," she said, "I used to have a front passage, and I used to have a back passage, but now I'm all a'one."

I examined her, as did my chief of surgery. What had taken place, 30 years before, was an injury that still occurs occasionally — the delivery had torn the outlet of the birth canal and had ripped the skin and mucosa all the way back into the rectum, opening up the rectum and tearing the circular muscle that enables us all to control bowel movements.

This significant injury, if recognized and treated immediately, can be corrected. Suture the rectal mucosa, join the torn ends of the circular muscle, repair the vaginal mucosa and the skin, and usually the mother is on her way home in a few days.

Not so for this patient from the Labrador coast. The well-intentioned granny probably recognized the problem but couldn't do anything about it, other than hope that the ripped mucosa, skin, and muscle would, by some miracle, grow back together again.

It hadn't. My patient related, sorrowfully, that she had no more children because "my husband would have nothing to do with me, that way."

This problem can occur in a hospital setting as well as elsewhere. In the hospital, however, the severity of the injury is recognized and the problem repaired. Most family doctors are trained to identify and treat it. I have done so. Certainly, general surgeons and especially obstetricians are well acquainted with dealing with this recognized complication of delivery.

Fast forward now: I'm on the North Shore of Conception Bay in 1969, in the middle of a bad winter. We have just suffered through a snowstorm, one of many that year. The main highway is open. The drungs are not.

At 2:00 a.m., a lady from Angashore Bight, thought to be eight months along in her first pregnancy, calls me.

"I'm havin' pains, Doctor."

Into the car, a little red Volkswagen, quickly, black bag in hand. Pitocin in there, if needed. Sterile gloves. Clamp for the cord. Ready for any eventuality, but hoping none of it is needed.

The main road is open. Some snow on the lower end of Ochre Pit Cove Pond. Wind northwest, blowing a gale down the pond. Blowing snow on the road. I get through.

I walk down the drung, up to my hips in snow, 200 yards to the house.

In labour. Pains still far apart, but definitely not false labour.

I can walk to the car, out on the highway. She can't.

I call the snowplow man. I know his number, right off. I had to call him the day before. Lives close by. Drung blocked. Mrs. —— in labour. Open the drung so I can get the car down. Ambulance gone to St. John's.

Ten minutes. Fifteen minutes. Jesus, what's goin' on. Twenty minutes. I call. He answers. I'm havin' a cup o' tea, he says. I can't get goin' without me cup o' tea, don't ya know.

I swear, under my breath, a foul oath. Don't want her to hear.

He arrives. Down the drung, blocked with snow. Fence posts going up in the air. Fence wire and longers. Can't tell where the edge of the path is, snow over everything. Who cares?

I examine her. Two fingers dilated; in good labour, well on. We'll make it to Carbonear. Don't you worry, missus.

Husband worried. Phone the hospital, I say. Tell them we're on the way. Half-hour, maybe.

Into the little red Volkswagen, and up the hill. No problem at the bottom of the pond. He just went through it with the plow. Twenty-five miles of gravel road to the hospital. We'll do it.

Pains every five minutes. Water intact. First baby, I say to myself. Thanks be to God.

Broad Cove. Doing OK. Getting there. Up through Kingston and around that loop of open country. Wild place. God help us if we go into the ditch. Delivered lots of babies before — 200, 300 maybe — in the hospital, never in the back of a Volkswagen in the middle of this god-damned winter, not on the road to Carbonear, no sir.

Up by the Barrens now, getting there, 10 miles to go to Carbonear hospital. How yer doin', missus? Pains every four minutes. Take it easy. Soon be there. Road in good shape.

Victoria. Long straight road, until the turn by the brook. Three miles to go. Up that hill past the brook. Goddamned hill. She won't go up. Slides back and forth. Ice under the wheels. Won't go up.

Pains every two minutes. Back down the hill. Give her another run, revved up. Up the bloody hill.

"I'm soakin' wet," she says. Water broke.

C'mon, car, get up to the top. Give her the gas, get up to the top. Aha! Up she goes. Over the top.

Wanting to push now. "I feels the head coming down." Missus, don't push, for Jesus' sake. We're almost there. Breathe hard, missus. Don't push. Soon be there. There you go, missus, we're goin' down Bennett's Hill. Turn left and we're there. "Don't push."

Aha. Past Harbour Rock Hill. Almost there. Never delivered a youngster in the back of a Volkswagen. Don't aim to now. Don't push, missus — see there's the hospital — don't push, missus.

Out they come. Waiting for us. Onto the stretcher. Away into the hospital she goes.

Jesus, I'm worse off than she is.

MOTHER MULLALY *of* *the* OBSTETRICS UNIT

SHE WAS BORN ON THE NORTH SHORE and, at the time of this story, was working as a nurse at a hospital close by. She was in her early 60s; she had been a nurse since the age of 20, and except for short periods when she took time off to have her three children, worked continuously at her profession.

The doctor met her when he worked for a short period at the same hospital. At that time, her duties were confined to the obstetrical department and the nursery, where she was head nurse, and where she worked for many years.

She was very religious; in regard to the obstetrical patients and their babies who came under her care, she spoke of them as God's creatures and treated them not only as a nurse but also as a mother. For this reason she was referred to as "mother," in much the same way as some nuns are called "mother so-and-so."

We will call her Mother Mullaly.

She was short, probably 5 feet 2 inches, and somewhat overweight. She wore her greying hair in a bun on the back of her head, which sometimes interfered with the wearing of the obligatory nurse's hat. In those days, nurses wore white, and each hat was distinctive, indicating the nursing school the nurse had attended. She wore a gold necklace with a cross around her neck, and on the front of her chest her nursing pin from St. Clare's Mercy Hospital.

She was a very competent and dedicated nurse and kept up on the latest techniques and ever-changing medications by reading nursing journals, and, as well, by learning from the young just-graduated nurses who came under her supervision. Her hours as a head nurse were pretty much as she chose, because of her seniority. Indeed, during the time the doctor worked with her, she never confined herself to any rigid schedule and could often be found on the wards at all hours. Her three children had grown up and left home, so she satisfied her mothering instinct within the confines of the hospital, which was situated close by her small house.

Many stories could be told about this remarkable woman. This is just one.

A young woman in premature labour came up from the North Shore. She was "seven months along the way," or 31 weeks gestation when her water broke, and several hours later her labour pains began.

Shortly afterwards, she delivered a boy, not much more than a pound in weight, so small that he could be held on the palm of an outstretched hand. He was a typical small scrawny premature, with no subcutaneous fat, so that his veins could easily be seen through the thin skin. At birth he had a strong cry, not at all like the high-pitched whine heard from very ill newborns, and he was moving all his limbs just as vigorously as if he were a full-term infant.

"And look," Mother Mullaly said, "look how strong his grip is on my little finger. You know, I think he's going to make it."

Still, the chances of this child surviving were small. Nowadays the child would be transported shortly after birth to an intensive-care neonatal unit with all the facilities and care of highly trained specialists. Back then, these infants were fed, kept warm in an incubator, given the best of nursing care, and everyone hoped for the best.

The infant certainly got the best of nursing care. Mother Mullaly took him under her wing, and it was good that she did. Shortly after birth, a recurrent problem began, which continued for three weeks. The child would suddenly develop episodes when he would stop breathing, often after periods when he appeared quite stable with healthy pink skin colour and good respirations. The monitor attached to the incubator would sound its warning, and the child would be found with no respiratory movements and blue skin colour, indicating a severe lack of oxygen.

Often the nursing efforts to get the child breathing again would be successful; often they were not, and the doctor, on duty or not, would be called. The child, on his arrival, would have skin that bordered more on black than blue; he would be "flat out," with no muscle movement anywhere on his body.

The doctor, having some anesthetic experience, would intubate the child. This involved under direct vision, through the mouth, of the opening of the wind pipe, inserting a tiny tube into that organ, sucking out the mucous with a suction apparatus, and then with a few puffs into the tube, the hoped-for result always occurred: the chest would rise with each puff of air, the blue colour would rapidly turn to pink, and the boy would begin to breathe again on his own.

Mother Mullaly, during that three-week period, spent more time in the hospital than out, and she was the one who invariably called the doctor when the problem occurred yet again.

The child needed to be intubated 20 times, and 20 more times the nurses were successful with their own efforts.

A lack of oxygen to the brain will invariably cause brain damage, especially if it is prolonged or recurrent. Once, in the middle of the night, having been called out of bed after the child had had multiple episodes as described, the doctor said, "Mother Mullaly, what are we doing this for? What is the point of it all? You know what's going to happen here. We're going to end up with a severely brain-damaged child, a vegetable. That is, if he makes it at all."

She looked at him. She was just as tired of it as he was. But she wasn't giving up.

"Ah, Doctor, we've got to do our best. After all, he's a child of God."

Shortly after that, the episodes stopped occurring, and from then on the child thrived. He began to put on weight and could be taken out of the incubator for short periods so his mother could hold and bond with him.

The weeks and months went by. Five months after birth, the child went down home to the North Shore.

He grew up to be a normal, intelligent child. When he

was in high school he won a mathematics contest that had entries from all across Canada.

Years later, while doing a locum back on the North Shore, the doctor met him and told him the whole story, details of which, up to that time, he was unaware.

"You are alive today," he was told, "not because of me but because of the care you received from Mother Mullaly and her nurses. I played a part but she was the main cog in the wheel."

It was suggested that since, at the time, she was still alive, in a nursing home, he could go and meet her.

It would certainly have made her day. It would have made her proud and thankful.

She died, however, before the meeting could take place. Greater love than this, no man hath.

ACKNOWLEDGEMENTS

THIS BOOK WOULD NOT HAVE BEEN POSSIBLE without significant input from family members — especially from my wife Florence-Ann, who was persistent in her encouragement when my spirits flagged, and from my daughter, Katherine, who did yeoman work in preparing the manuscript and offering advice and encouragement. My thanks go to them and, as well, my sons Craig and James Patrick, who proofread and corrected, and my sister Rosaleen, who researched the family tree of our grandmother, to whom the book is dedicated. Also thanks to my brother Fabian, a scuba diver of note, who filled me in on the extent of the sandy bottom of Northern Bay harbour, a significant factor in the great disaster of 1775.

Last but not least, thanks to Heather Crossman, the initial typist, a student at Oulton College in Moncton at the time of the writing of this book, who had to deal with page after page of my handwriting.

ABOUT *the* AUTHOR

WILLIAM O'FLAHERTY was born in Northern Bay, on the north shore of Conception Bay, Newfoundland. He completed an undergraduate degree at the University of Prince Edward Island — where he was editor of the college magazine — and a medical degree at McGill. After seven years in family practice in St. John's, in 1967 Dr. O'Flaherty returned to Northern Bay to begin his career as a country doctor. In 1989, he continued his work in Blackville, New Brunswick, on the north shore of one of the main branches of the Miramichi River, until retiring in 2000. Now retired, he lives in Moncton. Dr. O'Flaherty is a member of the Writers Federation of New Brunswick.